ETHICS

OF

HEALTH

CARE

Dilemmas of Technology
and Technique
in Health Care
and Psychotherapy

Edited by
Henry L Lennard
Suzanne Crowhurst Lennard

GONDOLIER PRESS

ETHICS OF HEALTH CARE
Edited by: Henry L. Lennard and
            Suzanne H. Crowhurst Lennard

Typed by Karen Bird, Boulder, Colorado

GONDOLIER PRESS, Box 467, Woodstock, N.Y. 12498

Library of Congress Catalog Card Number 79-57022
International Standard Book Number ISBN 0-935824-01-4

The Conference on Dilemmas in Health Care and Psychotherapy was held under the auspices of the Center for Policy Research and its Director, Amitai Etizioni. I am grateful to the Center's Administrator, Clara Shapiro, for her cooperation. The organization of the Conference was assisted by a grant in aid from the William T. Grant Foundation. I am deeply indebted to the former President of the Foundation, Philip Sapir, for his continued interest and support.

There are many of us who have benefitted from Phil's counsel, support and friendship over the years, first during his tenure at NIMH and subsequently at the William T. Grant Foundation. This book is dedicated to him!

Henry L. Lennard

TABLE OF CONTENTS

PART IV.

Note: All of the Conference presentations - with one
exception - are included, but some exchanges among
participants and audience have been omitted. Page
numbers for the presentations include discussion
as well. (For information on format see p. 171.)

INTRODUCTION

Lawrence Durrell [1] complimented Freud on his intellectual daring in treating "all human behaviour as a symptom".

Professionals have increasingly tended to conceive of human beings as patients. The extent to which this view pervades Western culture is well documented. [2] In first announcing the Conference under the title Man as Patient: What Price Treatment, I hoped to call attention to where we were, and what it may cost us. For salvation from psychological deviance -- the modern equivalence of sin -- comes at a high price. [3]

Technology and Technique: R.K. Merton in his introduction to Jacques Ellul's The Technological Society [4] tells us that Ellul uses the term technique to mean "far more than machine technology. Technique refers to a complex of standardized means for attaining a predetermined result". I share Ellul's view in conceiving of technology and technique as a continuum, both essential to a technological civilization, a civilization that in Merton's words is "committed to the quest of continually improved means to carelessly examined ends". Hardware technology (biological, medical and nuclear) seems to present more immediate ethical problems and responsibilities than does the use of therapeutic techniques. However, the acceptance, if not worship, of technique in one realm of social life serves to reinforce its acceptance in other realms!

To emphasize this very interconnectedness of issues inherent both in the use of high (machine) technology and in social intervention techniques, I planned for us to be concerned not only with major trends in medical practice -- using the development and application of highly potent psychoactive drugs as a case in point -- as well as with micro issues, that is, the increasing emphasis on technique in small-scale, face-to-face interventions, especially those applied in family psychotherapy.

---

[1] Lawrence Durrell, Monsieur, the Viking Press, New York, 1975.

[2] See, for example, Philip Rief, The Triumph of Therapeutic, Harper and Row Publ. New York, 1966.

[3] It is, of course, not the economic costs which I am referring to here.

[4] Jacques Ellul, The Technological Society, Vintage Press, (1964) p. vi.

While therapists and social scientists who view themselves as "humanists" are on the whole more sympathetic to a critical consideration of technology -- including that of medical technology -- than they would be of an examination of human intervention "techniques" -- they need to heed to F.R. Leavis' admonition that "the advance of science and technology means a human future of change so rapid and of such kinds, of tests and challenges so unprecedented, of decisions and possible non-decisions so momentous and insidious in their consequences, that mankind . . . will need to be in full intelligent possession of its full humanity".

One of the most important segments of medical technology, what has been triumphantly named the "pharmacological revolution", is a psychoactive-drug technology that significantly affects perhaps one-fourth of all persons living in Western countries at any one moment in time.

A wide array of potent biochemical agents have been synthesized. Since many drugs have been shown to be highly useful against some specific diseases, there has been great incentive to discover and promote drugs with equally "magical" powers against the host of personal and social ills characteristic of human existence.

Time and time again, we are alerted -- in all spheres of life -- to major "breakthroughs" and made to believe that technology will ultimately solve all problems, including those created by technology (such as toxic drug effects). An American scientist widely known for his cancer research is reported to have said that "We are on the threshold of engineering human cells so that none of the things we now call "disease" need exist at all".

Such "predictions" imply that suffering is indeed entirely avoidable and may result in a growing disinclination -- on the part of many -- to accept difference and distress as an essential part of human life. They promote a longing for the technological fix that will "put an end to our troubles". Psychoactive drugs may -- in the short run -- appear to be such medical breakthroughs, though they may very well, in the long run, diminish those characteristics most uniquely human (e.g.: variability, sensitivity).

A belief in "progress", Irv Zola notes, is "part and parcel of a series of a value orientation . . . an orientation of man over nature, including his own nature and biology. Thus there is no river that cannot be tamed, no mountain that cannot be levelled, no force of nature that cannot be harnessed, and no disease or symptom that cannot be cured or at least treated."

One aspect of such therapeutic optimism, whether in medicine or psychotherapy, is <u>denial</u> 5/ -- the denial that there are mysteries never to be fathomed and persons who, perhaps, cannot be "cured" -- at least not in terms of what is commonly understood by that term.

To resist cure, not to be "normal", that is, <u>not</u> to be like everyone else led -- in the not too distant past -- to the most incredible barbarites committed in the name of treatment. 6/ But it is the intractable, the person who <u>will</u> be different, who cannot be cured, that is still an irresistible attraction to the pharmaceutical industry and to the strategic family therapist. A promise of cure is always held out, and finds its "true believers", though sooner or later they will transfer their enthusiasm to another miracle drug or to another "new" therapy modality. But professionals and laymen alike need to be reassured continuously that something can and will be done; that we are indeed <u>in control</u> of the unique and the unpredictable. This paradigm and <u>its</u> expression in technological medicine invited Ivan Illich's 7/ allusion to "Hubris", the term used by the ancient Greeks to characterize man's presumption to aspire to the status of Gods. Yet, the philosopher Hans Jonas tells us that the power of technology forces a new dimension of responsibility on contemporary man. "Modern technology has introduced actions of such novel scale, objects and consequences that the framework of former ethics can no longer contain them . . . Take, for instance, as the first major change in the inherited picture, the critical vulnerability of nature to man's technological intervention -- unsuspected before it began to show itself in damage already done." 8/

I hoped that our discussions would reflect Jonas' challenge that the "new kind of intervention exceeds the old ethical categories. They have not equipped us to rule for

---

5/ I owe this insight as to the latent function of the "rush to treatment" to Otto Allen Will.
6/ See for instance, Emile Kraepelin, <u>One Hundred Years of Psychiatry</u>, The Citadel Press, New York (1962).
7/ Ivan Illich, <u>Medical Nemesis</u>, Calder and Boyars, Pub. 1975.
8/ Hans Jonas, <u>Technology and Responsibility: Reflections on the New Tasks of Ethics</u>, Social Research, Spring 1973.

example, on mental control by chemical means . . . undertaken, let us assume, for defensible and even laudable
aims. The mixture of beneficial and dangerous potentials
is obvious, but the lines are not easy to draw . . . 9/ If
the new nature of our acting then calls for a new ethics of
long-range responsibility, coextensive with the range of our
power, it calls in the name of that very responsibility also
for a new kind of humility -- a humility not like former
humility . . . but owing to the excessive magnitude of our
power which is in excess of our power to valuate and to
judge." 10/

Which Outcomes for Whom: Merton has observed that
"unanticipated and undesired consequences of purposive action . . . are less apt to mobilize pressure for preventive
or remedial measures than those problems that violate a pre-
vailing morality."

"Therapeutic" interventions, whether psychotherapy
or medical (surgery, drugs, radiation), have multiple consequences not only for the different organs and functions
of the individual treated, but also social consequences
for his family and other groups of which the patient is a
member. Some medical practices, in the service of a particular social policy (e.g.: treatment of addiction, mass
screening for diseases), often have far-reaching consequences for the life of the community as a whole.

Monitoring of the diverse outcomes of medical practices may well be necessary at a time of rapid application
of technologies capable of profoundly altering the quality
of life and experience of those to whom they are applied.
Not only need we attend to the problems created by such
dramatic advances as kidney dialysis, organ transplants and
in utero identification of genetic diseases, but also to the
moral and social consequences flowing from the most ordinary
medical practices, the use of drugs, radiation, and surgery.
A discussion of the multiple consequences of medical technology and practice for the individual, and especially the
family, was a major agendum for the conference.

Illness as a social phenomenon. Every medical action
has a social dimension; an impact on the patient's life and
on those for whom he is a significant person. Health-care

9/   Hans Jonas, ibid, p. 48.
10/ Hans Jonas, ibid, p. 51.

practices, therefore, involve personal and social values.

A conflict of values arises when the elimination or
control of disease becomes the ultimate or sole objective
of medical practice, though other goals and values may often
be more significant for the patient.

The philosopher of science Wartovsky reminds us that
"medical ontology recapitulates medical methodology" 11/
which I take to mean that the mode of treatment determines
the conception of the human being who is practiced on. The
physician's preoccupation with disease then obscures his
consideration of the patient as a person. Wartovsky states
this issue most clearly:

> The analytic abstractions of the human as
> a biological organism . . . leaves out what is
> most essential in differentiating the human as
> subject of medical practice . . . namely, the
> crucial . . . features of human sociality, human
> historicity, and the concomitant self-identifi-
> cation as human . . . 12/

The importance of the shift in emphasis became only
too clear when some years ago I interviewed an intelligent,
personable young woman who had spent four years of her life
in mental hospitals and halfway houses with the diagnosis
of "schizophrenia". She discussed her career as a patient
in a video-taped interview and her experiences with an array
of major psychotropic drugs prescribed for her over the years.
She described, most dramatically, the disabling impact of
the drugs on her physical, psychological and social functioning. Among drug effects she mentioned were lethargy,
somnambulance, lack of sexual feeling, memory loss, weight
gain, problems with vision and diminished taste sensation.

When I subsequently have shown the video-tape of this
interview to medical students to illustrate dysfunctional
side effects of psychotropic medication, considerable sympathy for the patient is evoked among the audience. Yet
after the conclusion of the interview, students routinely
comment this way: "The patient's experience is very moving
and arouses my sympathy, but would you tell us, please: Is
she better?"

11/ Max W. Wartovsky in Evaluation and Explanation in the
     Biomedical Sciences, ed. by Engelhardt and Spicker,
     D. Reidel Publishing Company, 1975.
12/ ibid, p. 67.

The students' question refers, of course, to the
status of the disease, of the "schizophrenia". It flows
from the assumption that drugs may affect the course of the
patient's disease for the better, though the patient's quality of life (as the students have just learned by viewing
the videotape) had obviously been greatly diminished.

The students' question illustrates vividly the dilemma that arises when the object of medical education and
theory is the disease and not the person. The task of the
healing professions -- and I can see no other rationale --
is to diminish distress in order that the patient's quality
of existence will be improved. Is it reasonable to claim
to "treat" disease when the therapeutic intervention results
in an over-all decrease in the quality of life of the person
so treated? Perhaps, high technology medicine has become
"autonomous" of the goals for which it has been developed? *

The Therapist-Patient Covenant: Analogous to the
development of a medicine -- increasingly technological and
powerful -- has been the trend to treat the canvas of human
troubles, foibles, and failures by an astonishing concatena-
tion of techniques applied by an ever-growing number of
therapists. What was once an enterprise limited to a small
number of persons -- for specific indications -- has become
infinitely expandable. Irrespective of the justification for
such a widening of "patienthood" ** and the number of persons
involved, the question that needs to be asked now, as it
might have been asked before, relates to the rules of human
conduct that apply to the therapist-patient transaction. With
the increasing awareness of "ethical" issues in medicine have
come occasional attempts to clarify these issues for the
psychotherapist and family therapy practitioner. These efforts, however, have been remarkably uninformed. In defense
of one mode of family treatment, use of systemic paradox in
family therapy, -- which raises issues of at least potential
violation of accepted rules of human conduct -- a well-known
practitioner notes "each person must come to term with it in
his or her own way". 13/ Haley, who should be credited for

---

* Gordon Allport's concept of "functional autonomy" may
apply to systems as well as to individuals.
** persons among whom may be many who, in the words of
Lady Macbeth's physician, are more in need of the
"divine than of the physician".
13/ Peggy Papp, Towards the Use of Systemic Paradox in
Family Therapy, (in press).

at least acknowledging the ethical issue in his writings,
comes to the remarkable conclusion that ethical obligations
are met when the practitioner provides competent help for
the problems agreed on, that is, fulfills the terms of the
business contract. 14/ In neither instance do the writers
appear aware of what has been traditionally and commonly
understood as the subject matter of ethics.

Therapy as a form of social activity is governed by
certain understandings that govern human relationships and
conduct generally, which cannot be abrogated or suspended
at will or unilaterally (except perhaps in the most extreme
circumstances and with the most extraordinary justification).

The Yale ethicist Paul Ramsey has perhaps given the
clearest statement on this issue, written with the physician
and medical researcher in mind, but no less applicable to
the non-medical therapist.

> "The moral requirements governing the
> relations of physicians to patients . . . are
> only a special case of the moral requirements
> governing any relations . . . between man and
> man. Canons of loyalty to patients . . . are
> simply particular manifestations of canons of
> loyalty of person to person generally . . .

> We are born within covenants of life with
> life. By nature, choice or need we live with
> our fellowmen in roles or relations. Therefore
> we must ask, what is the meaning of faithful-
> ness of one human being to another in every
> one of these relations? This is the ethical
> question (underlining is mine) . . . Justice,
> fairness, righteousness, faithfulness, canons
> of loyalty, the sanctity of life . . . are
> some of the names given to the moral quality
> of attitude and action owed to all men by any
> man who steps into a covenant with another
> man . . . " 15/

14/ "In therapy the ethical issue arises because the
     therapist is a humanitarian helping people who need
     him, while he is also making money on that help . . .
     to accept money and not give proper service in return
     is unethical . . ." J. Haley, Problem Solving Therapy,
     Harper-Row, 1976, p. 195.
15/ Paul Ramsey, The Patient as Person, Yale University
     Press, New Haven, 1970, p. XII - XIII.

If the therapist concurs with this position, then there are some questions he must ask of any modality he is using: Is its use -- in the name of therapy -- morally permissible? Does its use violate the "awesome" respect required of persons in their dealings with each other? What is the therapist's responsibility in disclosure and the giving of information to the patient or the family -- to keep the transaction fair and just? Is the patient's sanctity and dignity as a human being on a "common pilgrimage" safeguarded?

I wish to consider briefly how the covenant is safeguarded in the practice of "classical" psychoanalysis and in "strategic" family therapy, to make explicit the kinds of issues I take to have been neglected and to prepare the reader for their subsequent discussion during the conference.

The Case of Psychoanalysis: Persons entering psychoanalysis generally do so as a result of specific symptoms, failures of function, or as a result of diffuse dissatisfaction with their lives. In the course of analysis changes in behaviour, and outlook occur sometimes, including the reordering of value priorities and changes in religious or political convictions. There occur periods of emotional turmoil with the emergence of unsuspected and suppressed feelings.

Of course, all events triggered by the analytic process are subject to analysis by that process! Patients are also warned against acting out; against making major or irreversible life changes during analysis. Such injunctions, however, seemed more realistic in the early days of relatively brief treatment before analyses became as protracted as they often are nowadays.

The question arises whether the analyst, in not disclosing potential outcomes he anticipates, or know to be inevitable - does not commit a violation of the covenant or partnership with his patient. A further issue derives from the practice of excluding the patient's spouse, parents or children from participating in the initial treatment decision and contract, though they are intimately involved in the short and the long run. Not only are they profoundly affected by the daily vicissitudes -- by the ups and downs of the person in analytic treatment -- but, in the long run, analysis can conceivably be detrimental to their best interest though the outcome may well be in the best interest of the person in treatment.

Has psychoanalysis then been careless with concerning itself with the issue of informed consent and should attention be given to obtaining "informed consent" from the patient as well as from other family members? Should these significant outcomes for them - especially since not infrequently spouses and parents bear the financial burdens of treatment?

Significant arguments can, no doubt, be marshalled in opposition to routine disclosures to patients and relatives. But let us make explicit what these are and how they may be used in justifying what appears to be -- in the light of an emerging understanding of the professional's obligation -- a serious omission.

Family Therapy: Attention should also be drawn to serious issues posed by other therapeutic modalities, especially developments in the currently popular field of family therapy. I am referring to what has variously been called direct, strategic, structural, or paradoxical family treatment. To make what I take to be the ethical issue as clear as possible, I will not dispute the claims of those who practice in this fashion, that the strategies they employ indeed work -- and work with what they consider to be "intractable" patients and families. Consider the following excerpt from a description of the work of Milton Erickson, * perhaps the most widely acclaimed guru of strategic therapy. 16/ Erickson is quoted in the following abridged case description:

> "A woman in California wrote to me that her
> husband was totally paralyzed as the result of a
> stroke and could not talk. She asked if she could
> bring him to me . . .
>
> . . . I had my two sons carry the man into
> the house, and I took the woman into my office
> and talked with her. She said that her husband,
> a man in his fifties, had this stroke a year
> previously, and for that year he had been lying
> helpless in a ward bed in the hospital of a uni-
> versity. The staff would point out to students,

---

*   Though Erickson is not considered a family therapist, his "technique" has exerted great influence on leading family therapists, and consequently on their students.
16/ Milton Erickson quoted in J. Haley's Uncommon Therapy, W.W. Norton & Co., Inc., New York 1973, pp. 310 - 312.

in his presence, that he was a terminal
case, completely paralyzed, unable to talk,
and all that could be done was to maintain
his health until he eventually died.

I sat down in front of the man who was
helpless in the chair, unable to move anything
but his eyelids. I began to talk to him in a
roughly the following way. I said, 'So you're
a Prussian German. The stupid, God damn Nazis!
How incredibly stupid, conceited, ignorant, and
animal-like Prussian Germans are. They thought
they owned the world, they destroyed their own
country! What kind of epithets can you apply to
those horrible animals. They're really not fit
to live! The world would be better off if they
were used for fertilizer.'

The anger in his eyes was impressive to
see. I went on, 'You've been lying around on
charity, being fed, dressed, cared for, bathed,
toenails clipped. Who are you to merit anything?
You aren't even the equal of a mentally retarded
criminal Jew!' . . .

I don't know how he did it, but he managed
to get to his feet. He knocked his wife to one
side and he staggered out of the office . . . "

This is but one of many descriptions of the work of
Erickson where the therapist debases * the patient -- quite
unabashedly -- because he is, in his view, so clearly acting in the best interest of the patient. Similar examples
of the work of family therapist -- committed to strategic
and paradoxical interventions -- are freely provided in
their papers and lectures.

There is yet to appear a serious critique -- though
outraged comments can occasionally be heard in the hotel
corridors where papers describing such interventions are
given -- of the moral basis of such actions in the "name of
therapy". To act morally, Kant points out, one's actions
should be capable of being made the principle of universal
law. Moral principles are binding on all of us.

---

* Debase is defined by Merriam-Webster as implying
  "a loss of position, worth, value or dignity".

Entry into a therapeutic relationship does <u>not</u> carry an automatic waiver of these moral requirements. <u>The</u> moral intent or virtue of the therapist is not in question but as Jonsen and Hellegers point out, the ethicists' concern is with the "rightness of acts" not only with the "goodness of the agent". <u>17</u>/

Dilemmas revolving around the means-ends issue then appear equally significant for those concerned with health care technology as well as for those concerned with therapeutic techniques. The crucial question which we must come to terms with in both realms can be summarized as <u>Who</u> can do <u>What</u> to <u>Whom</u> in the name of <u>What</u>!

Henry L. Lennard
Woodstock, September 1979

<u>17</u>/ A.R. Jonsen and A.E. Hellegers "Conceptual
Foundations for an Ethics of Medical Care" in
<u>Ethics of Health Care</u>, National Academy of Science,
Washington, D.C., 1974.

PART ONE

Lennard: It is only fitting that a discussion of social and ethical issues
in health care and psychotherapies take place in a setting conducive to
leisurely talk, thoughtful interaction and human contact--such as Venice.

I am very pleased that it was possible to arrange this conference--
largely through the support of Mr. Philip Sapir, who is here with us today.

Let me now make some comments about what I take to be our focus,
though I do not wish to imply that we cannot change or restructure the
format of the conference along lines that we deem appropriate and useful.
I hope we shall ask questions not ordinarily asked and question assumptions
that have gone for too long unexamined and unchallenged.

Specifically, I am concerned with the unanticipated outcomes of technological developments: with the joining of science, medicine and business,
with a proliferation and adulation of technique--which is often indis-
tinguishable from technology in as far as technique does not allow for
spontaneity, improvisation, and sensitivity to individual differences.

It is necessary to think about these questions both in terms of the
health-care system as a whole, as well as in microsystem terms: that is,
in relation to our work with individuals and families.

Today I want to address myself to the broader, macro-issues.

Healing, whether it is the healing of physical or psychic ills, has become a major industry. In the United States, it is the third largest. The annual outlay for health care may reach two hundred billion dollars very shortly, and expenditures are growing more rapidly than in any other sector of the economy. Psychotherapies, and all other similar efforts at intervening in people's lives are proliferating. A character in a Lawrence Durrell novel says about Freud (and I paraphrase): "What a stroke of genius: to make all of human behaviour into a symptom!" And as a result, the image of Man as Patient now pervades our society!

Our attention is directed to consider such questions as: are we well or sick; normal or abnormal; too fat or too thin; is our family life healthy or disturbed and how can we tell? The media are saturated with programs about health and disease; witness the ubiquity of programs such as Dr. Welby, stories about hospitals, nurses, paramedics, and so on.

What does all of this mean? Part of the fascination stems from the remarkable developments in medicine, or rather in the basic sciences on which it is based (such as biochemistry, pharmacology, or genetics).

Part of it may be due to a loss of attachment to other systems of belief and support, the decline of traditional religion and other organized belief systems. Some have argued that "health" has become the secular religion, and that in the name of making us healthy, physically or mentally, we are permitted to violate all kinds of other values, to do almost anything to anyone, without fear of censure.

The health care effort as a whole seems to have become autonomous, detached from the purposes for which it is designed. Allport's concept of functional autonomy perhaps deserves mention here. Allport points out that some activities, perhaps initially undertaken to serve specific needs, later on become independent of those, and are continued for other reasons.

It appears to me that the medical effort, in its current manifestation, has become independent of the original purposes for which it was developed--to do something about disease in order to improve quality of life, to make us feel more comfortable! Often it appears that the massive machinery of medicine, once set in motion, with its specialized armies, special interest empires and agendas, proceeds to diagnose, treat, hospitalize, prescribe, instruct and interfere, without much concern about whether the consequences of these efforts increase or decrease the patient's comfort and pleasure in life.

Among the many issues we may want to consider is a set of problems ethicists write about who are concerned with the ethics of personal relationships in health care--with the physician-patient, experimenter-subject, therapist-client relationship. A position I find attractive is that there are basic covenants among men--and that every relationship situation (whether professional or not) is only a special case of the more general human encounter, and is therefore governed by these moral principles. The question arises: Under what conditions, if any, and under what circumstances may we suspend the obligations we owe our fellow men?

The question has many ramifications. For example, can a physician or therapist withhold information, deceive, mislead? And if so, under what circumstances? These issues do not seem trivial to me, because they concern the ways in which people relate to and treat each other.[1]

Another important issue arises from medicine and medical institutions being involved in society's failures--in assuming responsibility for, and managing the deviant, the addict, the difficult child, the impoverished, the delinquent. It is a role medicine has traditionally accepted--and even embraced--in redefining social as medical ills: on the one hand, to extend its empire; on the other, to provide legitimacy for the use of needed but scarce resources.

In a sense, medicine and especially psychiatry may be viewed as engaged in "covering up" the wounds and scars inevitably inflicted on persons and groups in a world where man and nature do not give equal justice to all.

A word about the new medical technologies--such as drug treatment of mental disorders: as treatment they are unspecific but may be used to deny that there are still unsolved mysteries, to deny the painful fact that we may need to live with other persons who construct their experience differently from the way we do, and who will always be fragile, vulnerable, in trouble, and troublesome.

The more potent technological tools (drugs, shock treatment) are a means to stifle the more extreme manifestations of difference; they function to permit us _not_ to listen or attend to the much more difficult task of sharing our social universe with those who perceive, and act differently from us.

Thank you. We will now hear from John Seeley who will also make some brief introductory remarks.

Seeley: I suppose that it's not unnatural that a body, gathered here, of friends who have known each other with varying degrees of intimacy, would have a very substantial overlap of perception, a very substantial identity of concerns, and even, whether by accidental or deliberate plagiarism, even ways of stating the problem. So I find it very difficult to follow after Henry--particularly as there was a very great element of surprise in my speaking at all at length this morning--without repeating much of what he's said.

I'll add two minor glosses: one, designed to expand slightly on the perspective from one of his statements; and one, in part to correct or balance, and thereby raise a very interesting question about, one of them.

Lennard is correct, I think, in stating that almost nothing is more popular on American TV than programs about health. In Los Angeles we have twenty or forty minutes of Health Hot-Line in the middle of the new "fun" news. But I must remind you that second, equal, coordinate and connected, is an equal obsession with the police--with the discovery of crime, the enactment of violence, deciding who is good or bad, and the elimination of enough of the bad to make it exciting without ever eliminating enough of the bad that the program would be discontinued.

This, I think, in both cases is the very pattern of what it is to be in this kind of enterprise.

I am even going to take a chance on reading (given the element of surprise) part of a paper that was written in another connection, because I want to make it as clear as possible what I mean by "being in an industry that has more in common with other industries than it has distinct about it." I want to make that particularly pointed.

Some of the things that I would like to add to what Henry said, if they are not already implicit (these are hasty jottings from the last five minutes), is that BROADLY speaking, as I see it, there is no real connection between the question of how to be healthy, and a quite different question--though the terminology used, the words used, are identical-- how to fight "diseases." We talk of the "health-care-delivery-system" when we mean "the disease-partial-counter-attack-support-and-maintenance-system." There is very little connection between anything that one could call a health enterprise and an attack on disease. And just as, in the same way, the suppression of vice (whatever that may be) has little or nothing to do with the enhancement of virtue, neither is it clear that the increasing mounting of attacks upon diseases has much to do with the institution and enhancement of health. I would have to add to that diseases, whatever they may be, are indefinitely expansible; that is, even if you "conquer" (if that is what you aim at) rather than maintain. If you nearly wipe out bubonic plague, all that does, immediately and obviously, through the whole length of history, and wherever you look-- is to permit you the luxury of attending to three other, and perhaps more

esoteric, interesting, complicated, perhaps not so brutal, but certainly
engaging and interesting, diseases. So that the model--which was the
whole progressive model in knowledge, of there being a finite realm to
conquer, and that as you moved out, like the navigators mapping the globe,
labelling and conquering and populating and civilizing one terra incognita
after another, that somehow there was some end to that--is a completely
false metaphor. What we are engaged in is something much more like a
voyage into space, where, as the horizon expands the sheer number of
points on it, and breaches in it permits a continuing, endless expansion;
every increase in the size of the circumference produces an identification of elements that do not conform to expected or desired patterns--
which we will then be pleased to call "diseases."

Put it another way, something more familiar--it is a form like
consumerism. The notion, perhaps even as late as our own childhood,
was that the conquest of poverty would occur as people got more real
income, more material goods, better houses, cleaner water, whatever.
Except at the margin which, as far as possible we keep excluded from our
consciousness, that is where there is real and bitter poverty in the
third world and the ghetto, but in our own lives that is not the case.
When we have a house that has four rooms, that is poverty because five
rooms is what is needed. And when we have five rooms it would be a
house with a better view, or nearer the sea, or whatever. So the sense
of poverty, or of deprivation aggrandizes with what was thought to be
the conquest of poverty. The problem of health is basically in that

model. A much better metaphor is that of the limitless horizon where the
circumference endlessly expands.

I would also draw your attention (these are just ad hoc remarks) to
how oddly drawn the notion cf disease is. It is drawn from some kind of
more or less flexible conception of biology. It is obvious that if you
have a broken arm, you are functioning in some way that is not quite as
desirable as if the arm is functioning the way you expect it normally to
do. This notion of disease is drawn from biology (and in its more fancy
and affluent form, from what we are pleased to call "psychology") which
by some false drawing of lines, or some convenient drawing of lines, is
taken to mean something that goes on in some sense, a sense that I don't
quite understand, in the interior of us and that doesn't appear subjective
that isn't defined as something having to do with organ systems and tracts
and ligaments and nerve connections. But to restrict what we mean by
disease to those two fields, and to leave them formally unconnected with
the--in both senses of the word--much more serious problems of moral
misery: how to exist in the world where, unless we keep it sharply out
of consciousness, we have so much while so many have so little, is
strange and arbitrary.

How do we keep out of the realm of disease imaginative impoverishment which is partly an accomplishment, partly a consequence, partly a
result of technology itself? How do we keep out of the realm of disease
the deterioration of political life so that in the really serious sense
we cannot be said to be any longer political persons or political
animals at all? How do we keep out of the realm of disease the diminution

of warranted pride, of orientation, of a sense of where we are or what
we are in the universe, the world we really inhabit, our only one and
real home. None of these gets labelled as disease, though on any formal
basis one would suggest that they have at least an equal, and perhaps a
better, and certainly a prior claim.

Finally, like everything else, anything through which so much money
flows as flows through "health care," becomes an Industry; and, as you
well know, the object of an industry is, if not to expand as far as
possible imperialistically, once that is no longer possible (though I'm
not sure we are out of that stage yet), it is at least to assure its own
stability and continuity. So whatever we call "health," or the "disease
fighting enterprise," becomes primarily an industry with odd people like
us who, for the most part, constitute a marginally permitted, but dependent entrepreneurial substrate. That is, like a petit-bourgeois surround
to the ITT and ATT of our own field. We are allowed to run Mom and Pop
enterprises of our own which partly satisfy our consciences, but in so
operating go to stabilize the system.

Insofar as that is the case--I hold it as almost (minor qualifica-
tions apart) wholly the case--all ethical decisions (the subject of this
conference), all major ethical decisions about matters that matter, are
thereby preempted, except that we are also in what Rieff calls a sort
of remissory enterprise, permitted to waste further time by discussing
the marginalia and trivia of the ethical problems of our industry, such
as whether or not we should deceive our patients--a much-debated question--
and the degree to which we should exploit them, psychologically in terms

of other kinds of satisfaction, financially, or otherwise.

I am going to read now a passage from a paper. The point that I want to make from it, whether you agree with the details of it, or not—and I hope what I say may affect the conference at least in part—is that a great deal of what we will be struggling with has very little to do with whether we are good and well-intending people or not, and a great deal to do with the structures in which we are embedded. The occasion for this paper was a very recent conference on seemingly the very lofty level of Prevention in the Field of Alcoholism. This was the summing-up paper. I am breaking here into the middle of it:

. . .When X, a very capable, strong, and sensitive woman—when X in a genuine cri de coeur—asked "But what are we trying to prevent, or do?" I said at the time, I did not believe we were trying to prevent or do anything, except, perhaps, very comfortably to survive. And further, that whatever we might think we were doing or preventing, what we were acting in, consciously or not, willingly or not, was not preventing something, but acting in (the Government's own words) a "prevention scheme"— which is a very different scheme than anything remotely likely to prevent what it is formally said to be intended to prevent. We are no more intended to prevent whatever it is (and I would like you to make the changes, mutatis mutandis from this narrow field to the foregoing), we are no more intended to prevent whatever it is (and even that is not clearly focused, in the sense of removing or radically reducing or abating it), than the police are intended to prevent crime, or doctors are to prevent disease. We are to maintain a preventive effort; that is, to carry on a moderated and controlled warfare against those given the means, subsidized, and aided by essentially the same employer to maintain the warfare, also without victory, so that an essentially diversionary spectacle (diverting both in the sense of entertaining, and in the sense of displacing effort from what matters to what doesn't) may be maintained, go through its variants, an analogue of a TV cops-and-robbers show, that will provide vicarious thrills, intellectual and good-against-evil dramatic, provide communiques and dispatches, and hills captured and valleys lost, but never, never win or lose the war. (Unless some higher order of necessity, which contributes to more important interests, should decree otherwise.) The view that something else is afoot, that is, that we are engaged in something else, that we should be allowed to do, or conceive, or propagandize for something that would be really effective, depends on a radical misunderstanding of what is a social problem, what, in a different vocabulary gets to be "accredited as" (and thereby becomes) a social problem: such as alcoholism or "substance-misuse" or delinquency or crime, or in this case, a "health-care-delivery-system." In an entrepreneurial, industrial, bureaucratic society, as I've often said elsewhere, and as must be obvious, nothing can be, or is accredited as a social problem that cannot, as one criterion, bring into being and maintain on an adequate scale, at least six interconnected industries. Firstly, there has to be an industry that creates, maintains, and, within limits, expands the problem. An organized crime industry, for instance, a distilling industry, a drug industry, a mystification industry called "school"; a sufficiently effective psychogenetic organization of work and everyday life, whatever you will--the problem-producers.

A second and a third industry must be called out, and these have to be elaborated as, ostensibly, a "hard" and a "soft" police, or counterforce, industry, suitably matched and adjusted to maintain the problem at just the right level of prevalence and incidence. (Incidentally, that almost invariably turns out to be five percent, whether it's delinquency, mental retardation, whatever you like. When it gets beyond that, you adjust the definition or the statute; and when it gets below it you do the same until you are back to about five percent.)

The hard police system is normally the recognized police and the hard-nosed professionals (such as some teachers and psychiatrists who act punitively in the place of the police, or who reinforce them). But there has to be also a soft police industry to divide the victims further, and to institute, in effect, out in the society, a graded minimum-to-maximum security system. This consists of non-hard-nosed professionals, such as most psychiatrists, psychologists, social workers, nurses, counselors, acting in their one kind of punishment-remissory character and recruiting out of the consumers for the industry those whose public service is to demonstrate, by going along with this game, by compliance, that is, by showing that they "need help."

The fourth indispensable industry, to help explain away the otherwise incomprehensible, completely organized, deadlock, is the research industry, which aims, it says, to try to uncover what the previous industries and their sponsors have set in motion and covered up.*

---

*Though, of course, they are never allowed to uncover the game completely.

The fifth major industry that must be made inaugurable is an education, or education-plus-propaganda, industry that carries the contentions of all parties, suitably mixed and balanced into a cacophony that has insidious effects of its own, but primarily into a mystificational system. This industry again permits shifting about in particulars (that is, allows guerrilla and tactical sorties, turning this way and that, while leaving the problem substantially as it is, except now further indurated by convincing those so educated of its complexity and intractability, or, with equal effectiveness, but falsely, of its simplicity--except for the machinations of some unreachable and unnamed bad guys).

The sixth necessary party or industry is a major industry of entertainment and communication to market the several cops-and-robbers games, so we can watch TV and ask ourselves, "Will the cops catch the little pushers? Will the psychologists spot, capture and save the potentially contrite? Will the researchers find and at least identify, if not indict, the noxious agent?"--and the high entertainment and gratification of the hunt, the capture, the trial and the punishment which spices our daily lives with vicariously enjoyed cruelty. Will they catch them, and, if so, what will they do with them, and who will succeed them, and how will the hunt go on?

I hardly need to add as a separate industry the bureaucrats, think-tanks, cabinets, or other coordinators, who facilitate this permanent play. I have to emphasize permanent, for note that the durability of the problem, or, preferably, perdurability (that is permanence, that is problem-insolubility), is of the essence and must be built in at the beginning, or provided by elaborate negative feedback. No such industries as I have described can be mounted, just practically, for a war of _brief_ duration--you do not call out the Army to settle a skirmish. People need tenure and career expectations in every one of the industries involved, and that requires problem-stability at least, and problem-expansion along inbuilt imperialist lines if possible.

I can't fill in here the variety of ways in which duration, if possible permanence, is assured to the problem. The ideal way is by stating it in insoluble terms (as I believe is true in the case of mental retardation). An alternative safeguard is to organize the industry _across_ problems, like a conglomerate, so that we ensure that persons with problems simply escape from one problem category into another, basically on an exchange system: prisoners go into mental hospitals (after a lot of work); mental hospital patients become community mental health center clients (after a lot of work); the center's outpatients become alcoholics or addicts; the latter cease being alcoholics or addicts, and become hypertensives or child abusers, or stroke or suicide or accident victims whom we "cure"--simply to put into another statistical category.

And note that, at every transfer point, as with a transaction- or sales-tax, the employer of all ultimately, that is the State, counts coups, and counts each transfer a success--an alcoholic cured, a prisoner non-recidivic--a sort of social-psychological gross national product.

Note, also, that as with a fixed supply of money, even if the transactions can be merely speeded up, the apparent psychological or social

problem solution income per annum--what the government takes credit for
and what we take credit for--increases. The finer we make the categorization of problems, the more rapidly we can increase this specious but
apparent income--indefinitely.

I want it to be clear, as I said before, that no matter how good
our intent (and I don't wish to make friends feel bad) our role in the
play as a whole cannot even faintly resemble our good intent. If it
did, we should collapse the enterprise that supports us, defeat the
State's interest, and collapse the society as we know it. As things are,
we are largely agents in, and as necessary to it as any of the other
parties to the overall game, which has as utility, on one side, the
stabilization of the system as a whole, and on the other side, the
recruitment into mutually defeating warfare, in the service of all the
parties involved, of the brightest, the best and most committed, who,
were they not so diverted and thus "otherwise engaged," would seriously
threaten the very foundations of the whole system, even if only by
gaining an adequate understanding of it, gained from and feeding into
a very different kind of praxis.

I don't know--if you are listening any longer--how to tell you how
to go from here, or what are the implications. But it is obvious, at
least to me, that nothing at all can be done without a clear and continuing recognition of the role that we play, our complicity thus in
the perpetuation of the problems we purport to deal with, and thus our
role as stabilizers of the growing social order--or, at the very least,

of such marginal changes as it is willing to make on the principle of the minimum feasible ransom.

I want to make one more point now and then I'll let go. The point is, my conviction is, obviously not original.

1. The summation of innumerable partial critiques, which is the danger we are likely to fall into here, is not the same as, or in any way similar to a critique of the whole system.

2. Only a critique of the whole gives us an appropriate point of departure, that is a warrantable foundation, for a non-trivial critique of anything that is part of the whole.

3. That, absent a critique of the whole, and a continuing institutional body to sustain the critique and the critics in it, there will be no such global critique, and hence no warrantable partial critiques.

4. Absent such a critique, we increasingly fragment life, rob it of meaning, and hence of the sense that anything is intelligibly better or worse, while claiming that that is the cause rather than the consequence of our hypo-critical stance.

5. Only in the search, single heart and single mind, for such a critique, will the dialectical process proceed, in which theory and praxis form and inform each other, and the critique enters as a circumstance both into circumstance itself and into criticism per se.

<u>Lennard</u>:

One of the panelists has devoted many years to studies in one area
of the new health care technology, the development and use of psychoactive drugs--and especially their use for women. We shall now hear
from my friend and colleague, Ruth Cooperstock, from Toronto, Canada.

<u>Cooperstock</u>: I have been working on the nature of the use of mood-
altering drugs and the meaning of that use, and more recently, particularly, I have studied the meaning of that use, as perceived by users--
in a very open, if you like, ethnomethodological, way. Henry and I
have done some of these studies together.

Let me make some general comments first. One of the things about
drug use today, and I am using drugs in the broadest sense--<u>all</u> drugs--
is that use on a worldwide basis is expanding so rapidly that we cannot
even begin to assess it. So the idea of disease as being infinitely
expandable is even more applicable to drug use--which indeed appears
infinitely expandable.

Prescription drug use is increasing ten to fifteen percent per
year on a worldwide basis. We have to ask: What is the meaning of
this trend? Is it related to the occurrence of illness? It is
perfectly obvious that the use is expanding most rapidly in those countries where the population is healthiest: in the Western world. A
number of very obvious moral and ethical issues arise, given this knowledge.

What are the problems of drug safety? We all know about Thalidomide and what happened. We know that five percent of the people entering medical and surgical wards of hospitals in the United States and Canada and Ireland and Finland are entering because of reactions to drugs that they have taken, or are entering on account of other iatrogenic complications. The issue is: Whose responsibility is it to protect the public from the consequences of drugs in their lives? Whose responsibility is it to protect the most vulnerable parts of the public? And, in this sense, on a worldwide basis, it becomes the Third World that we are talking about, where drugs that are no longer considered safe, drugs that are out of date and are no longer saleable in the United States are being dumped. This has been extremely well-documented recently in various publications. These are the places where one can go into a pharmacy and buy virtually anything over the counter. Whose responsibility, then, is it? There are few laws in these countries to protect their populations.

Turning now to the countries that most of us come from, whose responsibility is it to protect the vulnerable parts of our own populations? And, particularly, now what about psychotropic drugs, and tranquilizers, sleeping medications, the mind-altering substances that we are all very acutely aware of and that represent one-fifth to one-fourth of all the drugs that are consumed?

These high-use populations, we usually find, are the elderly, the institutionalized, the hospitalized, those in nursing homes, prisoners, young children, and, especially, women.

These are some of the issues that I am interested in, and I hope some of you are. One of the things that we are beginning to learn is that when we ask people why they are using these medications and what their effects are, they are defining and responding in terms of their social world. . . . And this is one of the fascinating things that we are learning from the work that we are doing. We set up small groups of people who have been using, or are currently using, tranquilizers, and we simply tossed out the questions: "What effects have these drugs had on you and your family? How do others in the family perceive you differently? How do you perceive your role(s) differently? How is your life different from before? How has drug use affected your relationships? How has it affected your work?" We simply got discussion going, and then we could just sit back and listen, because there was no need to do anything else; people got so excited being invited to express themselves in this area. We had a number of marvelously expressive and articulate people. One woman, who currently had five teen-age children and a rather demanding husband and a large house to look after, said, "I've used tranquilizers steadily for twelve years. I guess I use them to protect my family from my irritability." This was what they meant to her. This was how she perceived her world.

There are so many issues--neutralizing feelings, neutralizing roles, the way one can interact with one's world through the use of drugs--that one could discuss. I'm not going to go into it in any great detail here, but I hope we can talk about these issues later. I brought with me some transcripts of some of these interviews that we have done, and I think some of them are very moving and very meaningful. People have talked about why they use psychoactive drugs, why they quit using them, the consequences of their use in terms of their family, how the drugs have not allowed the individuals, particularly those with chronic illnesses, to express themselves within the family, how the drugs "get rid of" their feelings so that family members haven't known of or understood the feelings of these people with a chronic illness.

I was reading something recently, and it struck me very forcibly because it deals with the way one perceives oneself and the way one can alter one's own feelings. I thought I would read you this little quote:

> I have examined myself lately with more care than normally, and find that to deaden is not to calm the mind. Aiming at tranquility I almost destroyed all the energy of my soul, almost rooted out what finally is inestimable.

This has nothing to do with drugs since it was written in 1782, but it is a beautiful description of the perceived effects of tranquilization. It was written by Mary Wollstonecraft in her Declaration of the Rights of Women.

Sapir: Henry asked me as a representative of the William T. Grant Foundation which is sponsoring this Conference, to say a word of welcome and greeting to you, which I am glad to do. I am glad to be here too, for many and obvious reasons. I think it was very ingenious of Henry and his charming wife, Suzanne Crowhurst, to have this meeting here. We have a living, palpable example of a really fine level of human existence. I think that the many topics that Henry has listed in the program and that will be discussed during these days are very important.

And I hope something useful will come out of our meeting--useful for each of us. I started to jot down, as people were talking, little thoughts that occurred to me. And that's the fun of this kind of conference--every thought that one individual offers makes each of us, I suspect, have four or five of his own thoughts, of related interest and concern. And that's the value and the charm--and perhaps one of the dangers--of this sort of thing, because this is an incredibly broad series of concerns we have. I could just read some of the terms that I jotted down--"humanization"; problems of "medicalization," of "professionalism"; the "role of caring" in our society; the problems of our own personal attitude toward the professional, the healer, the curer, the magic medical man; the problem of the role of the professional man himself to his own curing, healing capacities; the all-powerful, all-knowing person who will give surcease to all of us; the problems of our social characteristics, what we do to each other when we get together in groups--and on and on. I could end up with a Panglossian prescription that all is for the best in the best of all possible worlds. I could end up thinking about our need for devils, and our need to beat them regularly and constantly, and so on. And so I will simply come back to my own means of maintaining stability--a thought--and that is: one may hope something useful will come out of this, such that each of us will think a little more clearly, or perhaps do things a little differently after we have thought over what has gone on in this meeting. And even if only a few of us do that, I think the meeting will have been a success.

And so, again, my thanks to Henry and Suzanne, and the others who agreed to come here and let us have a useful and interesting time. Thank you.

Lennard: Our next panelist too, is an old friend, Donald Bloch, the Director of the Ackerman Institute for Family Therapy. Don and I have known each other for many hears, and have many parallel interests.

Bloch: Thank you, Henry. I really will severely limit my comments, mostly just to give you a chance to hear my voice (slightly amplified) because my sense, I think is along the lines of Phil's thoughts: that the best thing about a meeting of this sort is the chance for some leisurely getting to know each other. So I will consider this really as a way of introducing myself to you.

It occurs to me that one of the things that one should do if one wishes to have a young city grow up to become a Venice is to be clever enough to site oneself where the automobile cannot get. In a sense, if there is a morality connected with that, or at least a level of an approach to this problem that is in keeping with my personal style, it would be to try to find what the pragmatics of the problem are. I was a little dismayed when John finished his opening comments, and I asked him afterwards, "Where do we go?" After that, because I found myself feeling that not only was all lost, but even the one thing that I dimly clung to--namely the notion that private virtue might be salvation--I now discovered places me squarely among the foremost defenders of

iniquity--and I couldn't think of a worse place to be. So I am going
to leave there.

I want to say a little bit about what I mean about the pragmatics--
or at least some approach to this. What I am addressing myself to is:
What can we control in our lives? and, Is there some way we can organize
our own sphere of influence, in some fashion, to live better and do
better? And I am going to assume that there are ways to live better and
do better. And associated with that, ways to live worse and do worse.
I mentioned that it would be useful to grow up on a canal--if you are
a city. If you are a social institution, or if you happen to have some
control over one, it probably makes a difference, for example, how big
you are. That is, I think you have a choice over that, and some way to
control that. And therefore, on my list of things would be the issue
of being the right size. And I'd like to suggest the connection between
those characteristics of institutions and their function in moral and
ethical terms.

I think one can control the degree to which one is specialized or
generalized. And there is something about being a generalist, while
being a specialist, that is a feature of how we organize our relationship to each other, or how we organize our own work or our own institutions, that maybe allows us to be better people and to do better things
in this world.

I think there is something about our communication structure that
can be defined in pretty specific terms. For example, the nature of
the communication network through which information is passed, the

length of communication lines and the number of filters along that line.
The perimeter of the system is related to the communication links within
it, and some of the characteristics of that, in rather formal terms,
can, I think, be defined, and I think they are related to ethical issues.
I think we can talk some about power, legitimating our concern with
power, and the issues about how it is distributed and how it is trans-
mitted. My special area of interest is with families and the distribution
of power in families and transmission from generation to generation,
which is a key definable issue about families and other social institutions. And I think it says something about whether there are better
places for people to be or worse places for people to be. I won't go
on at great length about that. I would just like to indicate something
about how I think, and the level of my concern. I am very glad to be
here with you and I look forward to a good conference.

Seeley: I think it is a very unhappy situation in which the choices and
proclivities of people may be unnecessarily restricted, whether that is
in our own ghettoes or in China, or wherever it is. I think it is very
sad to have a system in which it is intrinsic to the system that, with
every gain the wants are multiplied, because that is the only way
the system can be kept intact. So that the minute--and I repeat--the
minute you have reasonably clean butter you must have twelve alternative, though marginally differentiated, spreads. To keep the system
going you must have something else and something else and something else.

I must remind you that _that_ view of human life could only be forced
at the point of a gun or the whip of necessity (as in the industrial
revolution in England where you either starved or you manufactured and
consumed in a never-ending circle), or in the colonies when relatively
unspoilt men would say, yes, it would be very nice to work for the new
masters and to have a decent bolt of cloth to clothe myself with, and
a little better food for my family, and even perhaps a little of the
white man's medicine, but then went back to the hut and stopped laboring
frantically eighteen hours a day, for the rest of life. The only solution was to impose a hut tax, which, if not paid, would lead either to
the capture of the village or the shooting of its head man. And it
wasn't that much different in Bavaria from what it was in North Africa.
The only way you could institute this system of boundless hunger,
whether it is in terms of what you define as comfort, or lack of
disease, or whatever, was to _create_ the insatiability--first enforce
it by force, and now, since we are much better psychologists (the
psychologists have either taught, or the industrialists have learnt
from us by indirection, so we serve them directly or indirectly), we
know how to create those hungers non-insidiously. But neither of those
is, I think, to be taken as a model; and somewhere in there the hidden
question is: What is that art of life in which you balance those
insatiable hungers, whether they are for health, prestige, whatever
they all are together, so that they do not explode you nor implode you,
but permit a way of life that gives you a sense of being a whole being
in a whole world? (I will return to that later.) So that you are not

moved into a series of endless paths that must, in the end, leave you
unsatisfied?

Bloch: I am not sure I disagree with it but I would like to challenge
it a little bit. Just simply in terms of walking through the streets
of Venice. What is so remarkable about this city is that you never know,
if you go down a path, where you are going to come out. The novelty,
visually, is extraordinary. Each little square is different from every
other square. None of them is symmetrical and regular; no road leads
where it should lead. You can't count on the fact that if you come upon
a canal that you can walk along that canal any place because you may be
blocked and have to go around.

What am I talking about? Why is this a delight to us? It is a
delight for the very reasons that you are attacking. It is novel, it
is unpredictable, it is an explosion of all kinds of innovative diver-
sity.

Seeley: Can I reply? I would think the historical foundation is wrong.
A very great part of the reason that Venice is as it is, is because
Venice was defeated and driven out of the mainstream of that entrepreneurial, conquistadorial path on which it was set. There was a change
in trade routes plus a double defeat on the mainland. Between the mainland and the pirates and the enemy at sea, Venice collapsed and had to
turn back on itself and find its own satisfactions on a much more modest
scale, and could no longer aspire to the same kind of domination that

leads to empire, endless expansion and so on. Following that defeat,
a way of life which you now recognize as comfortable, and in one sense
quaint--that is, its happiness for us is in one sense that it is out of
the way, that it is unlike the megalopolis of this age.

The second thing that you point to as its delight, and which it
can permit itself, is in part for that reason and in part because it
is supported by tourists, like us, who, drawing boundless bounty from
somewhere else bring it here to keep that life going. . . . Part of the
reason it is a delight is that it is not a thoroughfare, it is a remissory part, it is like what you are allowed to do when you go home after
your day's work and can listen to Bach and Vivaldi, instead of continuing in the logic of the system.

I share the delight. I share the beauty of the dead ends, the
endless surprises. But that came about partly because the Venetians
fought to the point almost of extinction. The near-defeat by Genoa was
a turning point. If there had been sufficient victories, then Venice
would be the Rome, if not the Berlin, of the Mediterranean world. But
defeated, turning back, the Doge's palace becoming not the link between
the Byzantine Empire and the Europe it was imposing itself upon, it
could become a beautiful structure to be admired, sat before, lived,
entertained in front of.

Bloch: The other thing I wanted to ask is, Why are we here? and What
pleases us in this? And what pleases us in it is its variety and
novelty!!

von Trommel: You said what is admirable about Venice is the novelty. I think we are able to react to circumstances we have never met before, and I think one of the reasons for stress is that many people can't react as well as others can to events they didn't see before. So I think for us it is a very nice place to be, but many people need guided tours. When they don't find a guided tour they are unhappy and sometimes they are sick or ill. I think we have to put up with them, on one side to help them, to be a guide, on the other side to help society, to bring back our information in order that people need less of a guide.

For me it is a problem how to work--individually, as a guide, or a leader. On the other side I think a big problem of illness is our structure of society, in which there are every day more possible choices. And the more you can choose, the more you can confuse.

Lennard: Let me pick up on this analogy. People who used to come to Venice, years ago, studied about Venice and visited here on their own. I don't know when the notion of the guided tour came into being. But there is an impoverishment of experience that happens to people who come here on a tour, because then they must fit into the technology of the airplane, and of the tourist industry. The tourist industry is indeed a nice parallel to the mental health industry. To the extent that one offers these tours, one reinforces the view that the only way to see Venice is as a part of a guided tour. So you do not permit yourself the discovery of any other way to do this. This example illustrates the dilemma of the expert, who, by being an expert, in a very crucial way makes us inexpert, foolish, unable to do things for ourselves. The better we "experts" are at our jobs, the worse everybody else believes himself or herself to be. Only to the extent that we become less expert, the more expert will other people be. That's a good parallel--the tour. There are dangers to offering tours!

Shands: Henry, it seems to me that the enormous charm of Venice to us, comparing it to New York City, is that if you go to a certain store in New York and look for it where it was four years ago, it is not there anymore. There's a new tower block there. If you go to see the Palace of somebody on the Grand Canal here, it has been there for four hundred years. So that the charm of Venice to us is a relative novelty within an incredible conformity and solidity and stability, which has to do, I am absolutely convinced, with the lack of power. This is a powerless city, which has become a fascinatingly beautiful museum. New York, on the other hand, is an incredibly powerful city which is rapidly deteriorating--maybe, in three hundred years, it will be a museum too.

But I think that these are metaphors of the civilization, and the problems that we get into, the problems that are fascinating in this conference, show that we are doing the very thing that I am talking about. We are expanding further into the notion of an infinitely discussable universe. And that seems to be one of the major problems we face. Every week, over my desk, I get a new bureaucratic demand, formulating a new policy of responding to a new set of restrictions, setting up new committees to do this, that, and the other thing. It is very hard on my own mental health--this incredible, incessant novelty of the bureaucratic demands, in the name of ethics, morality, regulation,

evaluation and all of these great things that we all believe in. It is
a fascinating paradox.

Seeley: I would not like the analysis of the guided tour to stop--I
think the analysis is right--at the development of the airplane and the
tourist industry. It makes only small differences which side of the
capitalist-noncapitalist world we are talking about. The processes of
centralization and aggrandizement, the collection of power in central
places, are all served by the same process that makes for the guided
tour, and therefore, in a sense, the homogenization of people, rather
than their heterogeneity, and especially their looking at things they
are directed to look at rather than at being left to wonder.

Even these tiny questions connect with the highest questions of the
nature of the political and economic order and the concentration of
power, the oligopolies and the international conglomerate corporations,
which are the new forms of the State. So I want to run all the way
from questions that agonize you properly in your private practice--when
you can do better and worse--to the way those chances are weighted by a
system in which it is much more difficult for you to exert power.

I want to add something else. I believe I am cynical enough to
believe it is no accident. At least as long ago as twenty or thirty
years ago when computers were dawning and their potencies were clear,
a great deal was known, particularly after Von Neumann, about what was
called input-overload and its consequences. You can take very simple
illustrations of what happens to a gifted pianist; all you have to do is

speed up the metronome (with an agreement from him that he will try to keep up with the metronome). First the grace notes disappear; and then he makes errors of notes; and then he skips bars. There is a whole set of ordered disorganization under that kind of just-temporal overload. The minute it became clear what "informational overload" is and will do, people in very high places started talking about input-overload as an alternative to, or complementary to, an increase in police power. But input-overload--that is, facing people with more choices than they could use; giving them more information than they could organize; passing more papers over their desk than they could use; appointing them to more committees than they could conscientiously live with, so that they would be, not destroyed, which would be too visible, but defunctionalized, made de-usable from within--was part of the armamentarium of stabilizing a system in which no radical change in the relative maldistribution of power and privilege would have to be engaged in, but the horrors of con-centration camps, guns, gas, could be diminished, while these more subtle methods were employed.

I don't want to dissever the mini-problems from the macro-problems. There is an order there to be perceived.

Namkin: I'm Sidney Namkin from New Jersey. I hear two levels here, and they are implied in what Seeley is saying now. We talk about helping a family live or function better, but on that level one doesn't really affect the problems that he is talking about in the sense of the overall structure of the society. And what we do, in a way, is to give the helping professions a rationale for "covering up" for the system, for undertaking these tasks, which the helping professions have readily accepted--that they could solve these social problems. So that, for example, you turn on TV and you see the news, and they bemoan the fact that in areas such as very depressed areas where there is no housing and there are no jobs, and there is a myriad of social problems--they bemoan the fact that they don't have enough mental health centers, as though that was really going to solve the problems that exist in this area. So the kind of things that you are talking about really are the kind of things that--they act as a seduction or as rationale for the helping professions to feel that they are doing something useful, but they are really not affecting the problems that he is talking about.

Bloch: I think you have put your finger on a point. I think I understand it though I don't know the answer to it. Two years ago I participated in a conference in Rome. My point was to introduce family therapy ideas--it was a teaching conference sponsored by a Rome institute. The conference split on this issue, defined there as whether or not we were a counter-revolutionary group fostering technique at the expense of social change. The spectrum in terms of Roman politics ran from left to left. The sponsors of the conference were all communists; there was no problem about that, but they were far too right wing for the group that was critiqueing the conference, and exactly along the lines that you have just described. This was a much more intense issue there because it in fact was, as you know, the political situation in Italy then, and now was one where these were things that one could really get a handle on--not just simply academic discussions. I don't know how to answer that question. It is a long-debated question in the political left. I can remember as a student, myself, that the argument was made in the same terms--that anybody who contributes in any fashion to ameliorating the ills of society is a counter-revolutionary, and I remember in college, hot debates going on just in those terms. That was thirty or forty years ago.

I am not persuaded by that. But I can't argue this in anything other than some human terms. I think we have to deal with it on all levels at all times and I would want to, for myself, include John Seeley's analysis, which continues a tradition that I know he began thirty years ago (in his writings that I read at that time). It seems to me we need to be informed on that level, but for us to fail to move on all levels would, I think, be wrong.

Lennard: Let me add some comments here. I think there is a different kind of split forming around these issues. One part of it has to do with the means-ends business; the division between those doctors, therapists or psychiatrists who believe they can use any means for good ends, versus those people who believe there are only ends, that you cannot do anything unethical or immoral for any reason, in the name of therapy. This appears to be one kind of split.

The other one is illustrated by an experience in Switzerland this summer. In Olten, near Zurich, they are building a new nuclear power plant, and though the Swiss are among the most peaceful people in the world, ten thousand of them marched on this power plant and clashed with the police, who used gas on the demonstrators. This clash occurred in Switzerland, where this kind of action was hitherto unknown.

It seems to me that there are two groups emerging which we may label roughly as technocrats and humanists--those who believe in science, technology, and progress, even though it may destroy and pollute the environment; and those who question what we are doing in the name of progress, who agree that we have to learn to live with this technology, but believe that we have gone too far and wonder how to stop. I think that kind of split is not really left-right, because in the so-called left countries they are going gung-ho on technology too. The French communist union leaders, for instance, want nothing more than to build more nuclear plants, no matter what the possibility of potential accidents. So it appears that a new kind of division is forming. John, how do you fit this into your analysis?

Seeley: The problems about which I am basically concerned are less aptly stated in political terms even if anybody can identify any longer and agree on what is left, or left-left, or left-center, or whatever. I think, as you stated, a preliminary statement might be that the technarchy, by which I mean a technology which in your terms has become autonomous (though that sounds like a praiseworthy term) has spun off, by what in psychology would be called a split, and has become itself a form of self-sustaining insanity, unlimited, versus something that is much more cosmological and attempts to take into account the universe, which we actually inhabit, which is not just a physical space but a moral space. That would be certainly one way to put it. I simply avoid the

term "humanist" because, at least in the American tradition, you introduce
another split between humanists and various kinds of "religionists"--and
I'm not sure that that was what was intended. But it certainly has something to do with what is common to the whole culture, whether left or
right, in which control for its own sake, an endless conquistadorial
expedition to control everything, even (whatever that may mean) ourselves,
or each other, seems to be the sole deified enterprise and which, of its
nature, can never be ended and can never yield satisfaction. Because
that which conquers is that which is conquered! Even on a formal logical
basis it is like committing oneself to a process of self enslavement.
The outcome cannot be happy whichever side wins.

PART TWO

Nagy:

Maybe we are most practical when we consider radical points of view.
But perhaps, also, what I have to say will be in a different dimension
than what I heard most of the time yesterday, though I would like to
think that that dimension--fourth or fifth or whatever--was intrinsic or
inherent in what I shall say. Let me throw out a couple of ideas that
might make this connection. Some of them have been described in my book,
Invisible Loyalties. Some of them have been more recently added.

One is the ethical-dynamic point of view. By this I mean that
ethics (now this is a relational concept of ethics; it's not a value
ethics; it's not the science of what is right, what is wrong, what value
priority you or I follow),simply states what is one of the fundamental
dynamics of human relationships. It is the ethics of mutual consideration,
the balance of fairness, following from consideration for your survival
and my survival at the same time. If you notice, it is immediately on
a different level than any psychology is. A psychology says--If I am
considerate, my superego structure might be this kind or that kind; or it
describes my consideration conflicts with my needs, my rationality, my
id, and so on; if I am altruistic, or selfish--this all has to do with
individual characteristics within the person. I am not talking about
that. I am talking about the sheer realistic fact of whether you survive,
or whether I survive, and how is the balance between the two of us. If
I am alone on a desert island, then I can be very thoughtful, and plant
more trees, or plants to eat, or build a hut so that I survive better,
so I am smarter; but that has nothing to do with relational ethics.

The moment another person comes to that island, then immediately relational ethics becomes an issue. Because the other person has to survive, and I have to survive; and if I eat more and he has nothing to eat, or if in my sleep he kills me so he can eat more, or if we jointly plan and agree and work together for joint survival. . .these all have ethical-balance considerations. Now it is both your survival and my survival; it's not just my rationality. It may be that my rationality is to kill you off in your sleep right from the beginning, and then I have more to eat and less to work; but at that point I go to one extreme--the genocide notion of relational ethics. The other side is balance--"Let's work out a system whereby if I work more, maybe I get more rice, or we define what is an equal distribution of work. . . ." At that point we are in the realm of balance of fairness, so we are dealing with relational ethics.

It is my suggestion that this is the fundamental structure of relationships of any kind, the underlying ethical dynamic, balance of fairness--how it stands, how two survivals are balanced. And survival is more than just physical survival. It means also all the things that are worth living for.

This leads me to the notion of "parentification." This is very complicated. It can be thought of as a transactional idea. Those of you who know Eric Berne or Sal Minuchin or any transactional students of relationships might say: a child could be made to behave like an adult, and the adults can thereby get some benefit of managerial contribution from the child, and the child is going to be deprived of childhood gratification, because the child becomes accountable for the parents' needs, in a way. This is a transactional happening in any family from time to time, where we make children service the needs of a parent.

But on the other hand, ethically, this becomes an issue at the point when it becomes genuine exploitation; when, really, I do not give the child what the child is entitled to, to the point where the child will pay in his development, in his becoming a parent, when his child will pay--with a kind of a life-long deprivation (again a psychological term). The idea of justice here suggests there is an entitlement to resent the world. The world which is now exploitative, and phony and corrupt gives the child not just psychological deprivation, but a genuine entitlement to hate the world. This is a different idea. Something has been done to the child that has not been done to you or to me. Hence the child is entitled to resent the world. It is not just his crazy fantasy; he is entitled.

So at that point we have built in an imbalance of justice into a human life. This is parentification. It is an ethical construct. It is not just a transactional construct. You can locate it. The child is either child-like or adult-like. You can restructure it. You can make the child child-like or adult-like. But if you look at it in terms of a justice dynamic, it can become a lasting exploitative input, which then makes the child actually entitled to be unfair--maybe to the next generation.

This is a very important idea about society. Unfortunately the nuclear family is a preoccupation of the Western World; the idea that the nuclear family is very good and very successful, is used to put down the extended family, which I think is also a necessity. But I think that, unfortunately, what happens (what I see, at least) is that children begin to be made accountable in invisible ways. To give security to young parents, which they are not now getting from the extended family, there is behavior that is like borrowing from the funds of the future. I see this as accounting for many social facts: the fantastic number of young girls who become pregnant between thirteen and seventeen, particularly in urban situations; the enormous increase in child beating; the drastic jeopardizing of school funds by communities like Philadelphia. And then, at some point, someone begins to say, "Well this is horrible; something has to be done." And at that point--through the child--society in a magical way is made into a parent; and somehow this is a way of obtaining security, in a magical way, of being parented, being straightened out. You are not alone out there. Because if you hurt children, then someone will respond--first your child, and then your child's child; and then society, who will be horrified by your cruelty. I think this is a very sad thing, and I think the process goes on on a large scale.

One more idea: loyalty as a structure of society. I think as we talked yesterday I felt this idea was a little bit missing. I think if we say "Americans this. . . ," or talk about Italy or Holland or Israel or Japan--any of the traditional nations that have existed for centuries and are embedded in a kind of organic development--I think we miss a major point. I think that American society has a lack of definition, of commitment, of loyalty commitment, which is, in contrast, embedded in a historic nation (a nation which has at least a thousand years of

continuous history). Ultimately, a sense of being Italian is a very basic
commitment. In America, I think this is the first question for me when
we talk about what is being done in society, when we ask: What is justice?
To me this is a question that should be answered. What is the frame of
reference for deep commitment to society? Who cares, who really cares,
about the nation as a whole? About all these people who are there? In
the same sense as people who are willing to sacrifice their lives if
necessary, or have an intrinsic investment and pride in their own group's
achievement? That level of deep commitment and loyalty is one that needs
to be defined, if there is such a level. Before I can see a national
system or a societal ethic being defined, we must have such commitment.
I don't think we can piece it together from what we know about the power
manipulations of any group--unions versus management, or political
parties--or from what we know about families, or religious groups. These
are all there, but the overall structure of society, I think, either has
or doesn't have that deep commitment.

The last point I want to make has to do with what I described in
the book as "multi-directional partiality." As I heard the question
yesterday, it was: Should we be revolutionaries? Should we look for
scapegoats? As a family therapist I teach everyone whom I can teach,
and one of the most difficult things about being a family therapist is
to overcome just this tendency. I think most of us as therapists (people
who usually do individual therapy) came into this field because of a
kind of deep commitment to side with the victims against the bad guys.
(Usually the bad guy is the parent or the grandparent or someone who is

"bad," or "old-fashioned," or so on.) That is deeply embedded in our own basic psychology, I think. So it is embedded also in society--that this group is bad; that is good. Yet real progress, I maintain, is not by a revolution which appoints the bad guys and chops their heads off and then supposes that everything will be fine. I think that the same system then re-establishes itself; just that the heads would be different heads.

I think real progress can only be made by a kind of multi-directional partiality. By this I mean not a lukewarm neutrality of not taking any positions; the opposite, I think--that sharp positions should be taken on the basis of convictions about what is good. But then the merit of some other convictions should first be looked upon from the viewpoint of inquiring: What is the merit of their position? We are Catholics in Ireland; what is the position of the Protestants? So if you can, you should come from a kind of multi-directional point of view, and try to put together what resources there are in any human structure; and, first, define the resources in any loyalty structure. The Basques are loyal to being Basque. This is annoying to us because we are Spanish. But let's look at what it is that they are willing to risk their life for, what are their values, what is it that holds them together for some construc-tive goals, and so on. And maybe there is a way to look then at our values and to begin to balance the resources in the two systems, rather than saying, "The more we ruin them the better for us"--which is the traditional attitude. Now we can say, "Let's use the resources from the different systems." I think this leads to a better understanding of what loyalty commitments are. If we say they are criminals because they

will blow our Prime Minister up, so they will look to us just like any
criminal who would shoot you for money--no different. Or we go over to
their side and see them as heroes who have to do this because there is no
other way, so that is the only way in the world to have power, to be
heard, to get somewhere, unfortunately. There is no way of negotiating.
The only way is to fight to the last; and we have to do the same thing if
we are to be boss. At this point, it is an interchangeable position--
their heroes and our heroes--but because they are _their_ heroes, they are
our criminals. And then we get into an invalid world in which we are
blocked from using resources.

So, coming back to relational ethics, my main concern is not with
illness; my main concern is with this broad matter that is common in
society--the disintegration of the social foundations of trustworthiness
on which children could base their growth. And I see a frightening scale
of escalating disintegration of society from generation to generation.
I believe that in restoring trustworthiness we have to define an ethical
balance of fairness. I believe that is the only basis of trustworthiness--
if there is some chance for fairness or for balance, if it is not all
power games and clever manipulation. But there is needed a definition
of what at least would be fair between groups, between families, between
parents and children--if there is some definition of that then I think
there is room for trustworthiness; and if there is trustworthiness, then
I think there is chance for trust in the sense in which Erikson uses the
term.

Audience: What might be said about the ethical tie between the healer and the patient from these perspectives? And perhaps we can carry that a little further along and think of it in terms of such social concerns as people who formerly were not patients being made into patients; or human behavior that was in other domains before being made into "sickness." Are there ways that these perspectives might inform that kind of consideration?

Nagy: Thanks for the very important question. It really leads, in my mind, to a certain definition of "contract." The ethics of the contract for treatment is radically different from the individual traditional one. Because, in my mind, the main contractor let's say, as between myself, and a patient or a family, is first and foremost the one whose life is going to be affected the most by my intervention. If my intervention is any good, and will have some effect on somebody, the person who will be affected the most fundamentally by my intervention is the main contractor. And this leads me, frequently, to the children--or the children's children, who are not even born yet. Because, as we know, the interlocking of generations is such that, if we help the parents successfully, then the children will benefit from it, and the children will more fundamentally build in the benefit into their future because they are in a vulnerable, early-developmental phase of their life. So, therefore, the impact of, let us say, a divorce (or no divorce) if there are small children is, in my mind, greater on the children than on the adults, even though, seemingly, you should consider marriage therapy versus divorce therapy. In my mind, the first matter to settle is: "OK. Now you people may or may not get a divorce. I would like to help you with that. But, in my mind, the main contractors, if there are small children, are your three-year-old, your five-year-old, your seven-year-old children. Now, can we first define what we all will do as a team, as making the best arrangement for the children. Now once we have formed a base for that, now I can hear how I could help you, and you, as a man and a woman."

Bloch: Does it follow from that that if a contract is poorly made, if the person who is affected has no power in making the contract, that that would in effect lead to an unethical position?

Nagy: I think that that is a sad conclusion. Because it would sound as if all individual strategy of therapy would either be inadvertently victimizing others, and callously being indifferent to them, which is unfortunately true with some of them; or it would fail to use the best leverages for health, because some of the best leverages for health are in the relational dynamics;

. . .So I don't know how to avoid that implicit accusation. I don't like it, and yet it is implicit in this kind of thinking.

Audience: I applaud your thinking, but it sort of implies there is an abundance of resources which will balance out, when in fact there isn't an abundance of resources, and people don't have the same abilities to negotiate, and so on. So it comes to the practicality that somebody usually takes a show of hands. And then I'd like to know what "entitled" means. Does someone end up with a credit that is going to be given to his children? It is a very rational idea, but why isn't the process happening?

Nagy: I think it requires a longer exposure to see how it really works in the therapeutic setting. Let me tell you this--it does not work, in my experience, without the therapist's conviction, which he can only gain by a slow absorption of what this means in his own relationships and in relationships he is working with. Again and again, one gets discouraged, and encouraged; and that is my experience with training. No question that this has to be the therapist's conviction and activity. It's a very active therapeutic attitude. For instance, I can say to a person, "Yes, I can hear you describe everything. It was horrible. You were rejected by your parents. When you were seven or eight they took you back. Then you found that two younger children who were born were not rejected. Then at just the point when you started to deal with your hostility to your parents (it so happened that this was a family victimized by Hitler) Hitler moved into that country and all your family were wiped out. So here you are. On the one hand, you hate your parents. On the other hand, they were victims and martyrs. On the one hand, you were deprived and you are entitled," and so on. So where do you go from there? There are situations in which it really is extremely difficult to find resources. Nonetheless, one of the basic principles is that the so-called dialectic of give-and-take has to be assumed to exist, an idea goes beyond the usual psychodynamic notion. The usual psychodynamic notion would be "Alright, this child is then deprived. So what can you do with it?" You sympathize with it, or you make the ex-deprived child desensitized to it, if he has the resources. It's a value function anyway. Then you go through a painful analysis: "Do you want to live or not? This is your past, so what can you do?" That would be a kind of ego-strengthening approach.

I would say there is one more thing. There is the child's deprivation because the child wanted to repay, and there was no means to do it because the parents behaved badly, and then the parents disappeared. So it is true the child was deprived because the child did not receive; but the child was also deprived because the child was deprived of the possibility of repaying. So therefore I begin to work as a therapist on that--that is a resource, that's a tremendous resource. "Now here you are, and what can _you_ do?" It's an active question. It's not: "How can we commiserate because you had such a wretched childhood?" That's a passive attitude.

But maybe I say, "Well maybe we can do some work on your parents' childhood; maybe at least we can exonerate them. Let's understand why they were such impossibly-behaving people. Do we know enough about their childhood? Let's find out, is there an old aunt alive. Why don't you go over there and find out about your parents' childhoods." At that point the patient begins to give to his parents who are deceased, who were bad parents, who deprived him, at least the beginning of advancing to them a kind of human, balanced, understanding. "You now want to humanize them instead of keeping them as monsters. You say, "Well, there must be a human explanation." At that point, you give to them, and you receive by giving. By making your parents more human you also receive. If you keep them as monsters, you deprive yourself still further. If you are able to give them back, by trying to understand them as human beings, at that point you also give to yourself.

Lennard: I find your views fascinating! Let me go back to something which you mentioned earlier, that you attempt to determine who is most affected by the intervention. That this has become a concern of yours. You are dealing with an important but general issue that may apply the interventions, whether chemotherapy or psychotherapy. Who is most affected by a medical or a therapeutic intervention? What would you do in a situation, one I have seen very often, where the contract is to deal with a child? Yes, it turns out, when I talk to the therapist, that he knows that the father is a cardiac patient or a diabetic, in very bad physical state, who may easily be physically disabled by any kind of aggravation. And yet when you say, "Who is dealing with the father?" who may be very much troubled by what happens in therapy, the therapist will say, "Well our contract in this clinic is to deal with kids." Now is there any way out of this? Is there any way of ordering values? Is there guidance one can give? Under what circumstances does one pay attention to whom? Does one say, "Well maybe given the circumstances the symptom of the child is not so bad." The hazards of treatment are too considerable!

Nagy: Again, the resource itself is in the relationship. This is a very hard translation. The resource is not in a kind of yet-unused brain cell or a yet-unused insight capability of the mind. That's a psychological notion of resource, that you hear: you connect things, you remember, and finally you put it together differently, and you begin to use that resource of insight. In my way of looking at it, the resource is in the relationship. For instance, that father would say, "Well I cannot afford to care about my child, my child is no good [supposing it is a delinquent child], and I can only worry about my health." The child would say, "My father is old-fashioned; he doesn't understand me." The first resource is in the therapist's conviction that the parent and the child in some basic way are connected, that one's survival, in a way, enriches the survival of the other, on some level. There may be many ways in which they have different life-interests, but the basic that the child's life doesn't just go down the drain is in the interest of the parent, no matter whether the parent says, "I don't care, I am indifferent. I hate my child." But on some level I just assume as a basic premise, that there is a shared survival interest there. Similarly, the other way around, the child will never live as happy if he feels that his father died believing that his own delinquency killed him. So he will be better off if this is bridged by something in which there can be a give and take. So this is the conviction of the therapist: that his job is to find an area where this could be worked out between the father and the son. And this is the resource.

Seeley: I promise not to divert the discussion to yesterday's level, because I want there to be a lot of departures coming from this level. But I think I want to enter one caveat, because I don't want the line of thought to be too far from my point of view. An idea surfaced yesterday--that whatever we mean by "revolutionary" is someone who is looking for bad guys and good guys. But it is really precisely the opposite.

That is such childish behavior, that nobody who seriously calls himself a revolutionary, or has begun to start down that path, would allow it to himself. As I keep on stating, the people who appear to be bad people are actually captives in a structure that they no more control than you control the universe. So to make the alternation between revolution and the discovery of mutual and common interests a polarity, is so to falsify the picture of what it is to be a revolutionary that it is either a serious error of terminology, or it creates a straw man. Above all, a revolutionary looks for the system--and not to the defects of particular human beings.

Nagy: Let me respond to that. I am not putting it on an individual basis. I am saying that even systems--that every system deserves the dignity of being a loyalty system. I am saying something different. I am saying that even the so-called bad system is, on another level, a beneficial system to those who have commitment to it. Now I'm not talking about mechanical systems that are purely bureaucratic. I am talking about commitment systems--that every commitment system should have the dignity of being explored for its merit. I'm talking about the ethics of systems.

Seeley: Then I'm sorry. Then I do have to disagree. When your leader is being tortured in a Brazilian or Chilean jail, it is an inopportune moment to consider deeply the internal loyalties among the torturers--which are undoubtedly there, and which at some marginal point merit respect-- especially if by disregarding that for the moment, you can rescue the victim from the electrode applied to the genitals. I don't want to lose sight of that perspective either.

Anderson: We shall now hear from Dr. Harley Shands.

Shands: What I would like to tell you is a sort of a detective story. It is a report of about ten to twelve years of trying to understand something about a particular syndrome of de-humanization which I fell into quite by accident, and purely in terms of a profit-seeking motive on my own part.

I was designated (quite by accident as far as I was concerned) as an impartial specialist for the Workmen's Compensation Bureau in New York. The problem that I am confronted with in that role is to decide whether or not the disability states that people complain of are causally related to a particular accident occurring in the course of their occupation.

When I first got this assignment I had never seen a claimant, I had no contact with these problems, and I was a little bit astonished to be designated as a specially qualified physician in the role of the "impartial specialist" which is the way the law describes it. But I soon came to the conclusion that a lot of the people in the business were probably less qualified than I was, so that made me feel somewhat better about it. I have seen now about 150 claimants over ten or twelve years. Selection process is by no means random: I see people only after they have gone through perhaps two to eight psychiatrists, as well as orthopedists, neurologists, internists, and so on, who are looking for a specific definition of the syndrome which they present. In spite of the repetitive kind of selection process, somehow or other in the people I see, around two-thirds tend to present a syndrome which is internally consistent.

They come in and they complain primarily of pain, limitation of motion and a kind of vague malaise. Interestingly enough, for a person who used to be an internist, one of the curious correlates of this is that patients say that symptoms are worse in bad weather, which is a typical correlative of organic arthritis.

The reason they come to me is because they have been cleared by a specialist from any suspicion that they may have any kind of physical disorder. Many of these specialists--orthopedists, neurologists, orthopsychiatrists, write in the record: "This man has no organic disease; therefore, he is capable of working." The notion that they are psychologically or personality-wise completely disorganized is an idea that has not yet been accepted by most physicians in the United States, if this is an adequate sample.

When one really begins to do some kind of inventory of the distress that the people have--because they are very poorly equipped to present these symptoms themselves and they have to be specifically sought--the symptoms included, primarily, an amazing dehumanization. The complaint that they primarily make is that they have lost interest. Nothing is of any interest to them anymore; they are not committed to anything, they don't go to church or school, they don't go to play cards with their chums like they used to. They don't even to go the movies. One man told me that he takes his children to the park and he used to play with them, and now he doesn't play with them anymore, he watches them play. He takes them to the movies but he doesn't go into the movies with them.

He parks them at the door and waits outside and picks them up when they leave.

Some of these people even report (and this may be un-American) that they are not even interested in the television. Most of them report no interest in reading and the most astonishing thing to me is that when I asked them, "What in the hell do you do all day?" that question has no meaning to them. They don't know what I am talking about. They say, "What do you mean, 'what to I do all day?'"

Mostly they report complete lack of sexual desire. They report having become impotent or frigid. It is really remarkable. It is a complete wipe-out of everything one regards as a personality.

I began to ask them questions about the self, since it appeared that many of these persons did not have a describable "self" concept at all. But it is possible to map out a lesion in the self by asking questions. When I do, they routinely say: "Well, it's just not me anymore. Not myself any longer. I don't know this person, this person is an alien." Curiously enough, when the neurologist examines them closely, about half of these people have the characteristic "glove" or "stocking" type of hysteria--hyposthesia or anaesthesia of a half of the body or a particular extremity.

Again, it is very fascinating because most of these people don't know that they are numb, and to talk about "malingering" is a very interesting point when the person does not know he is hyposthetic or anaesthetic in a particular area.

Further, as a sort of comment upon unconscious thinking, it is obvious that the hyposthesia follows a cognitive map, but a totally unconscious cognitive map. It does not follow the distribution of the nerves at all. It is laid down rather than coming from the basic architecture of the nervous system.

Still further, my astonishment became extreme when I discovered that in these people there is no such thing (in most of them) as a neurotic prehistory. These people have never had a neurotic symptom in their lives. They don't have any idea what I am talking about. They are totally unable to describe anxiety. They are totally unable to describe feeling. If one asks a person of this sort, "Are you depressed?" the routine answer is, "Sure I'm depressed." And so I say, "Well, how does it feel to be depressed?" and the person says, "Well, how would anybody feel if they were depressed?"

One young man had a remarkable, astonishing paralyzed arm for two years. He had held it so immobile that it was sweating, blue, red, it was emacerated, it was a disgusting-looking arm. He told me that his mother had to help him dress (he was 21 years old), and so I said, "How does your mother feel about that?" and he said, "How would anybody's mother feel if their son was in this state?" The total avoidance of the first person pronoun is one of the most remarkable kinds of manifestations of this position.

The clue that has turned out to be most interesting turned up very early but I didn't realize that it was of any significance. Doing my standard psychiatric bit, I ran through a brief mental status and I discovered (it is reported in the second report) that these people were unable to tell me what is alike about an apple and a banana. That may sound like a simple and ridiculous item, but it is a clue in my detective story. The typical answer was: "Nothing is alike about an apple and a banana--an apple is round and red, and a banana is long and yellow."

"What is alike about a dog and a lion?" "Nothing is alike about a dog and a lion. A lion is fierce--and I am a dog-lover, myself. We have a poodle and it got clipped the other day, and it really did look a little bit like a lion." This is an incredible concretization, personification, individualization of the particular instance.

It wasn't until years after I began fooling around with this that it suddenly became clear to me that this inability on their part is a very significant inability because it is an inability to deal with the logic of classes. In the Piegetian schedule, this means that these people are pre-operational, which means that their cognitive development corresponds to that of a seven-year-old Swiss child. It means that the whole notion of conservation on which Western education is built is missing in these people--and that is really a stunning fact.

When I discovered that, it became a good deal clearer. In the first paper we wrote, we called this the "Freud-Charcot Syndrome." It was really a hysterical syndrome discovered and described by Charcot, and it is male hysteria par excellence. Freud is said to have astonished people by finding that males too had hysteria. But in this series, with

the pathognomonic sign of the "stocking-glove hyposthesia," there were five
males to every three females. This is a totally different sample from the
kind of people that one sees in the therapeutic context.

This became considerably more interesting a few months ago when
Bogin, the "split-brain" investigator from Los Angeles, reported that in
his work he had gone out and become acquainted with the Hopi--the Indians
from whom Worf made his original observations, and, to his surprise, the
Hope can't do similarities, either. So what that suggests very strongly
is that the whole structure of Aristotelian logic that we take as truth
indicative is an artifact of formal schooling. This has been a more and
more astonishing observation to me and it suggests that this syndrome is
characteristic of uncivilized people, undeveloped people, but it does not
occur in undeveloped nations. It does not occur among the Hopi--it only
occurs in an industrialized nation, and apparently it really began as an
interesting problem to pursue when railroads began to be common in Europe
In Ellenberger's "The History of the Unconscious," he points out that one
of the immediate correlates of the emergence of the railroad was the
emergence of railway spine, which, as far as I can tell, correlates highly
with backlash in legal procedures in the United States.

In the series that I have seen, most of these clients are unskilled
workers--about a half of them are immigrants; a large proportion are
blacks from the deep South with a similarly poor education; and something
like a quarter of them have required interpreters to be interviewed,
although they may have lived in the United States for ten, fifteen,
twenty years; they still can't speak English well enough to be interviewe

I was working for a while in a project in which the director has a remarkably successful method of rehabilitating prison inmates by teaching them dramatics. It is a program called "Cell Block Theatre" in New York City. The director wanted me to do some psychiatric work with the peoples' group work and, as I was not very much surprised to discover, my own peculiar talents didn't fit very well into that, but I did try for a while.

One of the things that struck me very strongly was that two men, one Irish and one Italian, reported almost exactly the same comment about their fathers. They "found" each other in one group therapy session one day. Both of them had experienced that their father was a tyrant: everything had to fit him at home; all of the children had to be very respectful; dinner was when he demanded it and so forth. Each of the sons remembered that he had gone to work one day for his father the tyrant and been totally astonished at work to find that the father was very servile and subordinate and respectful and humble to the supervisor or the foreman. And this "the king in his own home" and the "peasant at work" had struck both of them.

The significance of this seems to be that the father got his power from the occupation and brought the money and the status home with him, where the money allowed him to perform this role, and it was the only place in which he could do this, and at the sime time he was not powerful at all at work. What seems to be one of the interesting correlates of this particular syndrome is that the person loses his occupational status in terms of the compensation procedure which takes over after what

is usually a trivial accident. In one case, a man lost half of a particular digit and he was hospitalized for two weeks. Most people who lose a
part of a digit would go to an emergency room and have it fixed up and
never spend a day in the hospital. But because of the peculiar structure
of investigation-treatment in the compensation process, these people
become unemployed. (There is now a very remarkable amount of literature
having to do with the pathogenic effect of unemployment.) In addition to
that, they become functions of a process which they are totally unable to
understand--none of these people can understand my function, for example.
They come to me and they say, "Doctor, I have been sick so long that a
famous specialist like you can't help me, I am sure"--the idea that I have
no interest in helping them in the role in which I am seeing them is
totally unavailable to them--they do not understand that. They cannot
understand the organizational structure in which a psychiatrist can
function as an expert. They are unable, in other words, to define the
situation in the same way that they are unable to define themselves. The
fascinating thing that comes in is that they, too, choose the definition
of disease as a method of solving this particular problem. Their idea
of a solution is magical: they say routinely, "Doctor, nobody has been
able to find the pinched nerve or the slipped vertebrae, or whatever it
is that is giving me this pain, but I know that somebody will one day."

This young man with the paralyzed hand had been seen by the most
famous hand surgeon in the United States, the man who is the "father" of
hand surgery. And he insisted on saying to me, "I don't need to see a

mind-doctor; I need to see a hand-doctor." And the fact that he had been seen by the leading expert had completely missed him.

Ultimately, much of this began to be somewhat more clarified to me by a very interesting book by Alex Inkeles and David Smith, called "Becoming Modern." In this book, they report, in the mode of the Bureau of Applied Social Research, a six-thousand-interview sample--a thousand people in each of six developing nations were studied in terms of definitions of "becoming modern." In it, the most fascinating things were the deprivations required to become modern. What they lay out in very clear terms is that to become modern, one must first get rid of the extended family; second, one must get rid of traditional religion; third, one must get rid of traditional politics, and adopt new modes of involving oneself in political items; fourth, one has to get rid of the traditional hierarchical differentiation between men and women which, no matter how unjust, is still a major support for self-definition as the basis of differentiation.

After having gotten rid of all of that, one has to generate a self-definition in abstract terms to support oneself. The only thing that is really left to the unskilled laborer is his occupation. When the unskilled laborer is removed from his occupation and put in a situation in which he is forced to come to a new definition of himself, he is actually unable to see that he is the same person--in some sense--as the person he was, and he says in this pathetic, unavailing and repetitive way, "Well, Doctor, I am just not the same person that I was. I don't know what has happened to me."

The thing that seems to me to be the cream of the jest in some sort of cosmic joke of a very tragic nature is that I am convinced that it is the process of compensating people for this kind of disability that generates the disability that it compensates people for. The more one compensates people, the more there is a contingency of reinforcement (as Skinner would say) that perpetuates and consolidates the disorder.

One of the negative signs that identifies these people is that when they come to me they are universally--as all of us are prone to be-- afflicted with cupidity and their only hope of getting compensation is by getting a psychiatric diagnosis from me. If I say to them, "Do you think it is at all possible that there is anything nervous or mental about your disorder?"--"Absolutely not, Doctor!" There has never been anything wrong with my mind. Absolutely there is nothing wrong. This is some kind of disease that nobody has yet discovered."

So what we wind up with is institutional iatrogenesis, with a pyramid of paradoxes. The thing that completely paralyses me is how to generate any kind of therapeutic intervention that might make any difference to these people at all.

Thank you,

Crowhurst-Lennard: I am an architect, so you may think that I am a little out of place at a conference with this topic, but I believe there are a number of important areas where the concerns of architecture and of the healing professions overlap. Many of the problems that exist in the thera- peutic professions or in the medical care world, exist also in the architectural profession.

In addition, I want to stress we are all users or consumers of the architectural profession's products. We all live and work and play in man-made environments, and we are always in some way influenced by our immediate physical environment; if not consciously, then unconsciously, we adapt to or rebel against our physical environment. And perhaps if we are adapting unconsciously, that would seem to suggest that we are all the more controlled by the buildings we are in.

There has been, over the past few decades, an increasing emphasis on technology and building systems; and this has led to an increasing pro- fessional mystification, very much as it has, I think, in medicine. We tend to assume that only professional architects and builders know how to construct buildings; therefore, we tend to leave more and more decisions to them.

Another trend in architecture, which is reflected also in the healing professions, is the increasing tendency for architects to make decisions for unknown others. An architect will accept a job to build two thousand apartments for people he does not know at all. He may even not know their cultural backgrounds, or the various life-styles which his buildings must accommodate.

As a result of these trends, we have seen the proliferation of a modern architectural style which tends to alienate, and separate and homogenize us. This tendency has been particularly strong in institutional buildings, especially in settings that are conceived to be therapeutic--hospitals and places for rehabilitation. And this brings me to another link with the concerns of the therapeutic professions.

For some years, I have visited and studied environments for rehabilitation, and looked at the effects that the buildings may be having on the social program that is housed by it. I have found that often the buildings work against the establishment of truly healing relationships. Hospitals tend to isolate people from each other, to increase the barriers between doctors and patients, and to reinforce the hierarchical role-structure within the hospital staff, instead of providing places which heighten one's sense of wellbeing or legitimate a caring relationship between healer and patient. Hospitals are designed only to accommodate a functional relationship between doctor and patient, who are further separated by the additional intermediate intrusion of physical or pharmacological technology. In that sense, the buildings themselves may be iatrogenic of malfunction.

I also teach architectural design to architecture students and to students in other fields, who are interested in taking some responsibility for their own physical environment, and wish to understand better how to create or adapt their environments to suit their own needs and life-styles.

I think what I am trying to do in architecture may parallel what some of you are trying to do in therapy, in that I am trying to establish more of a "self-help" model in architectural design. I believe that people can make most of the important design decisions for themselves. They can make decisions such as: how they want to live and relate with each other in a real situation; what kinds of relationships they want to have with their family members, with neighbors, with friends. All these decisions have architectural implications. You can use a clarification of your own life-style as a basis for deciding where walls should be, how rooms should relate to each other, how your entrance to your living environment should relate to your next-door neighbor, and so on.

I am trying to return the responsibility of designing the environment to the users of that environment. I have to assume therefore, first of all, that my students can do it, and that it is all right for them to make those decisions for themselves. But I build into this process a kind of insurance by stipulating that, "In order to design a good building for yourself, you must first of all focus very clearly on the people themselves--yourself, the people you are living with."

This method of teaching architectural design is very successful on a small scale, where a student has to design for himself and five or six people he cares about and knows very well--his own family or close friends. Working at that scale it is possible to design very successful and very exciting and very beautiful buildings.

But I am often asked by members of the architectural profession, "Can't you systematize that? Can't you draw out a set of rules, so we can apply it on a larger scale?" But this method is not indefinitely expandable into a set of theoretical rules--which is to its advantage. You have to consider in great detail the quality of life in your own immediate social circle and that cannot be abstracted and generalized.

All architecture is, all buildings are, really a metaphor for a way of seeing the world.

Conversely, every way of experiencing the world has a potential expression in architecture. It is possible to read architecture as a set of concrete manifestations of the way people interact with each other.

One needs only to compare the grid plan of most American cities with the plan of Venice, to see vividly how assumptions about the nature of interpersonal relationships become concretised in architecture.

The grid plan was a result of the belief that it was perfectly legitimate for a centralized bureaucracy to impose territorial configurations and boundary relationships between strangers settling the land. Not only was it considered unnecessary and irrelevant to take the natural topography or "spirit of place" (Durrell's phrase) into account but, once the land speculation race had started, it became impossible for communities to negotiate their mutual boundaries and relationships. We have come to accept this formalized abstract way of designing the environment.

All architectural technology is an extension of the same attitude to dividing up space and appointing boundaries. Because of the technology we have developed we can only build square or rectangular buildings. We can only divide up space in that way and it is an expression of our technology and of our belief in technology that we do that. This room we are in [the Sala Tommaseo in the Ateneo Veneto]--I don't know if you noticed-- but the walls are not parallel! If you start with a focus on people, then a very different kind of architecture results.

The labyrinthine plan of this city--Venice--is an expression of a very informal, emotional, irrationally-based set of communications between people. Of prime importance are immediate relationships between people, and these cannot be rigidly formalized. They are not based on any abstract hierarchical system; they are based on people's feelings about each other, and can be constantly modified and subtly adjusted, as relationships ebb and flow.

Shands: I keep finding a paradox in everything we are doing.

What you are talking about is the dehumanizing effect of laying down a grid and having 168 streets in one direction and 11 avenues in another direction; and you are contrasting and comparing it with Venice. Which, to use a metaphor of some ancient nature, "just growed like Topsy."

It seems to me what you are saying is that Venice is fascinating to all of us because it is a manifestation of an unconscious process, whereas designing a city like the upper part of New York City is rational and conscious.

Then, if that's the case, if you refer that to the psychoanalytic idea-system, and say that what we are trying to do is replace the unconscious by the conscious, then you are saying what we should do is replace Venice by New York; tear it down and make it rational. Isn't that some kind of a paradox?

Crowhurst-Lennard: I think we call Venice a product of the unconscious because these processes that are made manifest in the physical environment of Venice are those processes which perhaps in the modern world we have tended to push into the unconscious.

Shands: Do you think it was planned?

Crowhurst-Lennard: I don't want to replace New York by Venice. But what I think we can do is add to the richness of New York by learning a little about the richness of Venice. There is a way of combining one system with another.

Shands: I would agree with you that our city planners, most of whom are heavily infiltrated with architects, have managed to destroy most of the really human neighborhoods in Manhattan that used to be enormously supportive of their inhabitants, and replaced them by the monolithic avenue of high-rise structures down on Columbus Avenue, which I find monstrous. But, isn't planning necessarily oriented in that direction? And when we plan mental health services aren't we necessarily falling into the same trap?

Crowhurst-Lennard: Only if you use the word "planning" to mean "planning the system and then trying to fit everything and everybody in that system.

Bloch: I take that to be a focal issue. We might say that if there is a correspondence of inner and outer space, if they are each constantly in the process of aligning with each other, never fully congruent, yet always coming closer, then to the degree that we have the opportunity to plan how we live, the space we live in and the social systems we live in, there are some better or worse ways to do that. And it seems that the paradox clearly lies in planning the unplanned--in finding some way to arrive at creative chaos. It seems clear that this is a constant, flowing enter-prise which, once it is completed is already destroyed! So that if we can address ourselves to this, if we can find some way of building in disequilibrated components to all stable structures. . . . Coming back, to how to stay alive. . . . From my perspective, the problem is how to build in mad poets, paranoid sociologists, feedback systems that are both deviation-amplifying, without being destructive to the system and, at the same time, deviation-reducing, without being killing.

I find what Suzanne is talking about enormously congenial, a kind of ethical perspective.

Shands: Isn't what attracts us to Venice the fact that this has a stabil-ity of obsolescence for four hundred years?

Springer: You said any particular architecture corresponds to a world view, a Weltanschauung--a way of looking at life. The point is how to bring the philosophy of Venice to the philosophy of New York. A lot of architecture in Venice as in New York is an architecture of power. I see a lot of power in Venice; not only the charm. Perhaps the poverty in

Venice has a little more charming architecture than New York. It is more
charming than in Vienna too.

I don't know whether the poor live very well in Venice, any more
than generally in the Mediterranean world. The poor people seem to live
better, because of the older ghetto situation. There are better community
structures; there are small communities. It's a grown-old situation.
Here they can live with their poverty. That's what we can see, and it's
most fascinating. We see the picturesque past of it. It's not just here
in Italy, but this you can see in Northern Africa, in Morocco. . . . The
Americans and the Austrians, too, come to look at the beautiful poor
children and give them their dollars.

The Morocco people can live with their poverty and, therefore, we
do not have the impression of poverty in their villages, as you do have
in the much more modern power-oriented architecture. The inhuman modern
architecture cannot live with poverty, don't you think?

Crowhurst-Lennard: Venice was a powerful State at one point. And its
greatest architectural expression of its power is in its most symmetrical
buildings. Take this building! This was obviously built by a powerful
man, and he was able to organize a large number of people. He had control
over a large amount of space. But even so, he, for some reason or other,
was not quite able to build an absolutely regular building. There are
all kinds of little quirks in this building, which came about because he
had to adapt to his neighbor or to a canal or to a painter who decided
to add a little piece somewhere, or to a builder who decided it wouldn't

fit properly that way and adjusted the measurements to fit more snugly
into existing site conditions. The owner obviously was trying to achieve
symmetry, but he did not have absolute control.

Nagy: I don't want to lose Don's point about ethics. Power, you know,
is very easy and obvious in this. But where is the ethics perspective?
I am trying to connect her observations with my system. Being in Europe,
and having been raised in Europe, what comes to my mind is that there
is a loyalty to the past, which is the opposite of the modernistic idea
of getting rid of the extended family connections: forgetting origins,
the continuity, the political traditionalism, the man-woman relations,
the traditions and so on. And that means I finally am able to rid myself
of all the ethical ledgers according to which I would know who owes what
to whom, who is committed to what. It begins to be a pure power again,
a pure survival by money. By contrast, I spent a few days in Heidelberg
and I know Salzburg well.   There one sees the issue of real commitment
to continuity of the surrounding--such as not to put a skyscraper in the
middle of Venice, even if it would bring in a lot of tax dollars in revenue.
Most people would rather be loyal to the continuity of their Gestalt.

Lennard: The neglect to attend to the physical environment can indeed be
viewed as almost unethical. The physician who sees patients in hospitals
in offices which are inhuman, sterile places, but who lives in Scarsdale
in the most marvelous artistic home. . . . The universities which expose
kids to the most atrocious environments while the professors in their own
lives are so sensitive to every little detail. . . .

We say we are healers in a place--we are healing you, we care, we are concerned--and yet put people into a nightmare of physical space. It may be that not all people are equally sensitive to the built environment, or that we have been sensitive at some point in our lives and this was knocked out of us. It may, therefore, not be accidental that Suzanne is English and lived in Oxford, and that I lived in Austria. . . .

There is an interface here of the world of environment and of our activities which we ought to attend to. That is what I think Suzanne is saying--Be sensitive to this!

There is another interface--if I may go on just a little bit longer- and this is what has been called by Roz Lindheim, the "Medicalization of Space." Not only are hospitals inhuman places, but, because there is so much money in building hospitals--they are the biggest, most expensive buildings, so that most architects who are any good are building hospitals. The model of hospital space then influences all other buildings. The technology developed for hospitals invades other kinds of buildings. So that, in the United States, unfortunately, apartment buildings and schools and universities and factories look like hospitals.

Seeley: Could I add, again, that I don't think these things are accident. And while in one way I welcome, in another way I regret, the overtone of attempts to change ourselves, the idea that we should severally become more sensitive--not that I wish we wouldn't, you know. But it is crazy not to recognize that we have been trained to make these splits, in a society that has an interest in our having those kinds of splits; a socie where the workplace, the serious part of life, is conducted in an exemplary linear fashion which disregards everything but a narrowed goal and a most narrowed economical means to reach it; and that this should be symbolized as far as possible--except for little wealthy districts and pockets here for exceptions--in schools that look like prisons, and indeed resemble prisons in other ways, not excluding lavatory passes and so on.

That is an essential way in which you are trained for a purpose in order to maintain a system--it is not to be overlooked. That in order for that system not to topple completely of its own misery--for not everyone to feel proletarianized--a number of people like professors and people who attend these kinds of conferences, people like us, are given, almost like Marie Antoinette playing dairymaid, places out in the suburbs; only, the next morning, to return to those dens where we will labor in those narrowed rational terms.

This room--it's roughly in golden section. That was no accident: it _was_ a way of showing power by paying respect outside and in. But that was in another day, when that narrowing, which is the crux of the present civilization, and which will be the thing that it looks to me will topple it--when that was in emergence and not, as it is at the moment, in domination. How to turn that I don't know. It may be that something can be done by trying to sensitize and reform ourselves severally and the few people we reach. But that sounds to me like a handful of us trying to bail back the Adriatic with a sufficient number of buckets.

Shands: I want to pick up the point that Henry made so forcibly. Most of us here are immigrants--I am an immigrant from Mississippi. But to go from Mississippi to. . .is like going from here to New York City. So there is another paradox involved here because most of us are immigrants to America, who then emigrate to Venice to discuss these problems. And the total absence of any representives of the power structure who might have anything to do with changing the kinds of things we are telling them they should change, is to be noted.

Bloch: I would like to identify a couple of other issues in what Suzanne has just said. She spoke about consumer representation and about the teachers being users. And it is interesting that, in psychoanalysis and in family therapy, we teach, for example, by having our students be analytic patients, or by having our students be family therapy patients. An essential feature of the way in which we help them understand their work, and ourselves understand our work, is to understand ourselves as individual persons and as members of family systems. It may be there is a little tiny corner of light there. It is a movement that has begun to grow into other areas. The whole consumer movement as such does provide, I think, that kind of useful disequilibration I was alluding to before.

Crowhurst-Lennard: I also am very optimistic that a revolution of some kind will be at least partially possible by people starting with their own small-scale decisions, such as deciding to tear down a wall between two rooms, or rearrange the boundary-relations with neighbors. It has happened in the counter-culture, and it is now expanding into the middle classes, in such movements as the loft developments in New York City.

To return to an early point that Harley made about planning. . . .
Architects in the past, in planning a building, first of all sketched an
overall scheme with some suggestion as to how the building would look
from the outside, and a rough diagram of location of major areas; and
they would then work towards detailing the inside of the building, how
rooms and corridors would fit together, how large windows should be, so
that the drawing of the facade looked balanced. . .and they would try to
make everything fit into this overall concept that they had at the
beginning.

But what is now beginning to happen is that architects are beginning
to say we have to start with the details of how people live and interact
with each other, and if we begin with that, then the building will grow
as an expression of the people, and the whole completed design will be
an expression of the larger organization of the whole group. And there
is beginning to be a little less fear of the asymmetry that results from
this way of working, and a little more appreciation of the organic way in
which it may express an asymmetrical social structure.

But in every design each small part must be worked out first and must
be allowed its own natural structure, and then the parts must be fitted
together in the most natural way possible, and finally the whole emerges.
And for every new situation--you have to work those out every time.

Nagy: Let me make a few comments about the morning talk by Shands. I felt some statements of his really fitted into my framework very well, his comments about modernism. I never thought of it this way but it makes sense, that modernism means that people are expected to be cut off from all that they are loyal to. They are cutt off from extended family, from their ethnic background, from their usual political ways of alignment, so they are in a vacuum as regards continuity of loyalty. One is loyal to nothing. This is very much the same thing I was talking about in relation to American society. Some groups--Jewish, Japanese, etc.--resist this kind of vacuum more, but most groups, and eventually maybe all groups, suffer from a discontinuity of what they are loyal to, or what they historically would have been loyal to. To me this was very important, because as we were talking about context--to me the context is not so important as what I would term the 'discontinuity of legacy.'

That, of course, I also connected with the ideas on architecture. Ethical continuity would involve a strict ethical balance between knowing who I am obligated to. For instance, the continuous loyalty to nationhood is an ongoing obligation system. Let us say I am Dutch. In everyday life the Dutch are very much like the Americans, they are very much oriented to a better job or a better income. Now, in comes Hitler and suddenly declares that Holland doesn't deserve to be a nation. At that point many people begin to react to an obligation expectation which in everyday life hasn't been expressed. In that situation we see heroes who are working in the underground risking their lives. So the legacy of obligation to a loyalty definition of society is there even though it hasn't been shown because it is not called forth in the everyday situation. But if the situation is such historically that it calls for that kind of loyalty, then the resources for its manifestation are there. Then heroes emerge, and this goes contrary to their everyday business striving, where people want a nice house, a nice income and a nice life for their families. Now they risk all, including their lives.

Now I would like to define two different things. The one is family loyalty. And the other one is a larger legacy that occurs in many societies, or in parts of societies, such as in a particular religio-cultural loyalty. I am obliged to transmit it to my child so that this whole system doesn't die out. This is the legacy. Family loyalty is a person-to-person loyalty--me and my parents, or me and my brother, or me and my child--which is a different thing from this trans-generational loyalty legacy aspect. I think that the term "modern" really refers to the discontinuity of legacy.

In some way I also want to weave in the architecture into this because I feel that the house means something! If it is an old family house I am expected to maintain it. It becomes like a legacy to not let it die, because my grandfather lived there!

Lennard: Could I try to make a bridge back to the concept of loyalty in therapy, and see whether Ivan agrees with it? There is an emphasis in our culture in the United States to make "dependency" into a dirty word. Professionals try to make their patients independent and autonomous. They often encourage children to leave parents and to live by themselves.

Autonomy is valued. In cultures like Italy, Greece, in pre-industrial cultures generally, dependency is not a dirty word. I am using the concept of dependency quite analogous to that of loyalty, a sense of being able to call on people, the sense that they owe you something, and you owe something to them!

In relation to a particular group of persons I have been working with lately, that is chronically ill patients, this issue becomes significant. The patient who lives out of town who has to go to the hospital for radiation treatments will say, "It is going to be very difficult, I have no one to take me for chemotherapy or radiotherapy." Then I say, "Well, isn't there anybody?" And he says, "Yes, there is somebody, an aunt or an uncle who lives fifty miles away." And you say, "Well, why don't you phone them?" And they say, "Well, I can't call on them. Why should they put themselves out for me!"

I think there has been an enormous emphasis on independence, autonomy, doing things for yourself, by yourself, in industrial western societies, and this trend has undermined a sense of loyalty. If I understand you, we pay for this loss.

Nagy: I think that the premises are still not clear, and I have to push further for clarification. I make a further distinction--dependence is a psychological, and in my terms, a power category concept. Namely, it assumes that the effectiveness of living would require that I, the weak one, utilize your strength, or that I, the clever, exploitative one, hang onto you and succour off your energy, or something. These are dependence terms and as such they are psychological need, or power-related terms. Now I think there is an even dirtier word in our culture--ethics. That is really a taboo word. And for good reasons. My speculation about some of the reasons are--because the word has been corrupted in use that one using it either sounds old-fashioned or unsophisticated, or tricky--someone who would like to use it for manipulative purposes, as it has been used. You know, if I can put the label of some kind of ethical judgement on you, then I really gain a few points.

I think that in extended family systems, corrupt, hypocritical, ethical priorities were manipulated and young people were locked into them. And I think it was a valid rebellion that in moving to America, that one would give up this whole system of bishops, and grandfathers and kings and go to this huge country where there was some truth.

From my point of view, the power rebellion is a very different thing from discontinuity of the legacy which is an ethical concept, or the ledger, the bookkeeping of continuity of obligations. You can rebel power-wise and not discontinue an ethical ledger. You can transform the means of payment and not just simply deny that there is an ethical ledger. This is a very great difference. I really want to make this distinction.

Audience: I really miss your first point about ethics being a dirty word. For whom, and by what right, is it a dirty word? The American Psychological Association demands adherence to an ethical standard.

Nagy: I don't mean it in that sense. I mean ethics as an explanation of human behavior. I'm not talking about so-called professional ethics.

I'm talking about ethics as a determinative motivational explanation of behavior. That is not used.

Lennard: To me, value judgements are what we are made of, and represent a commitment to a certain way of life. I cannot demonstrate scientifically that it is better to live relating to people than to be zombified by drugs, but I think it is better! It is my value, and I have to stand by it. At some point society may decide everybody should be zonked out, but this will not change my position.

Nagy: I agree with that. What I am saying is that I would like to talk about a dynamic structure of relationships between people. It is a description of a dynamic between people. It is a relational dynamic. If I feel exploited, I cannot stand by hopelessly being exploited all the time so I cannot stay in that relationship. I either become sick, or I leave the relationship, or I kill myself, or I kill the other one.

Lennard: So you are proposing an explanatory system for what happens in a relationship, and explains both the sense of owing, and entitlement.

Audience: I think what I am hearing is that you, for instance, were talking about the absence of loyalty as a basic value in American life; you are talking about a marginal man, someone who has no place in a context of relationships, who has lost his old loyalties and who is left in some marginal status, where the individual cannot relate.

Nagy: I think that. When I came to America, there was an Anglo-Saxon definition of the country. The picture I got was that everybody will

sort of melt into that format in a few generations. I think that notion
has radically changed, partly due to the establishment of Israel, partly
due to the Black movement--I don't know what all the factors were, but
the whole notion has changed. That's my private view. The fact is that
two thousand years of nationhood is different from one, two or three
hundred years of nationhood. It is still an active immigration land
and it has been so for a long time. Here the only genuine ethnic group
would be the American Indians. So in that sense I think that the United
States has not formed as a historic nation that has held through horrible
wars or one or two thousand years of history, which has been conditioned
to be a sort of an extended family, as the European nations are.

Lennard: Would you agree that the psychoanalytic movement, especially
as it has been introduced into the United States, as it has been understood by professionals in the United States, may have contributed to
undermining the loyalty base in the family? In the sense that it stresses
one's own development.

Nagy: But that's the whole individualistic Western cultural trend--one
very much influenced by the Jeremy Bentham Utilitarian philosophy of
democracy.

Lennard: Could we begin to talk about the topic of tomorrow, which I have
called, "the ethics of intervention." I'd like your ideas on what may be
a very subtle point. We know that in the course of a psychoanalysis many
people get divorced. Does the analyst say at the beginning of the con-
tract--let's say he analyzes the wife--"Look, we are going to work with

each other, but I want you to know there are certain things which may happen," like a surgeon who, before he operates, may say, "this may happen" or "that may happen." Does the analyst say, "Well, as a result of our work together, you may change your politics, or your belief in Catholicism. Or there may be an impact on your family during the time that you are going to be analyzed. Because of the analytic phase you may be in, you may get very miserable; you may get angry with your parents. Later on you will forgive them, but you may have fights with them during the analysis." I don't think he ever says that. Does this pose a subtle ethical issue? The individual therapist, in his work with the patient, is certainly influencing the daily rhythm and pattern of everybody's lives, not only of his patient's life. Whatever happens during that hour then reverberates in the life of the patient. This is what I mean by the ethics of intervention. Should he point out, Ivan, that he is really interfering in the life of the family? Should he get the understanding of everybody else involved?

Nagy: Yes, but the two are linked, because he should say, "If I am successful, then I would assume that the other family members will also benefit because the individual is a better-functioning individual."

Lennard: That is not really the issue. Let's say the patient is doing well and in four years time everybody is going to be much better off. But during those four years there may be a lot of disturbance in the family. And some parents may be very upset that that young person was up to that point very peaceful, but suddenly makes all kinds of recriminations against them. As professionals, do we agree to consult with

everybody and make explicit these possibilities and alternatives? This
is the issue that I would like us to talk about. We need to say that
we may create all kinds of nuisance.

Springer: In the case of doing therapy with young people, adolescents,
one should speak to the parents and tell them that there can be a disturbance in the family. I don't think one should do it in the individual
treatment of one partner in a marriage because you have to give them the
chance to outgrow the relationship. This is not disturbance, I think.

Lennard: But let us say you have two people; the husband pays for the
analysis of the wife. During the analysis she gets terribly upset. As
a matter of fact she may leave him as a result of the analysis.
The point is, to what extent do we need to inform people of the possible
alternatives of therapy?

Nagy: Let's modify the question. I would say this, that rather than
indicating that, "You also have a need; I want to be available to all of
you if you need me. So you should know, I am willing to treat X, it's
all right with me if only this one comes," I would say to the husband,
"but I want you to know that all of you--your grandmother, your child--
all of you can turn to me and I am very interested in being of help to
all of you. If you all come, that's fine with me." This is not the same
thing as saying, "I can tell you that you will have the danger of divorce,"
but I can say that I am curious about helping everybody and about the
interlocking relationships. I can help everybody better if I know more
about everybody. Therefore I want to be available to help everybody

whenever they need it. I don't think there is much risk in this statement.

Springer: You are in a better position working with a family therapist than with the individual analyst. Because the patient of the individual analyst must trust his analyst that he will not give information to another person. That is an ethical question.

Nagy: But I am also saying to these people, "I am willing to see any individual, especially a young adolescent separately, and you have to trust me with the privacy of communication." So I think that that kind of family therapy where you always meet together and always share everything is not appropriate here--I am not that kind of family therapist--I am saying I can see you separately or two or three together. I respect privacy and I will only tell things if there is any benefit, and you have to trust me for that. So in that way the ethics of confidentiality is handled.

Lennard: What is your obligation to other people whom you affect by your intervention without their say-so, knowledge or agreement? You are affecting their lives and they have not given their consent for you to do so. It is easier to see in other areas of medicine. It is an issue which psychotherapists have not dealt with so far, which they have not been willing to deal with. I suspect very soon they will have to deal with it. What is our obligation if we prescribe drugs to one family member--let's say the mother--we may also be interfering with the mothering, with the parenting relationship, etc. What is our obligation towards the other members of the family?

Audience: Supposing a woman comes to me wishing to enter into a contract for psychotherapy and I follow your course and I say, "Well, you bring your husband in on this as well, it is something that has possible consequences for him too." And he comes in and says, "No way, under no circumstances do I wish you to see my wife; I like the relationship as it is and I don't want you to touch that relationship, I want you to desist." The person who has come to me has been the wife. She is an individual. I assume she is an independent person, and I accept her right to come for therapy.

Lennard: That's fine, the alternatives have been pointed out now, the husband has said, "No, I will not pay for it." He said, "I think this will make life very difficult for us." She said, "It is going to make life very difficult, but I do want to enter this contract." What do you do under these circumstances?

I had a colleague who died of cancer. He and his physician made all the decisions about what needed to be done. He had chemotherapy, his hair fell out, all kinds of terrible physical things happened. The wife knew nothing about it; she saw all of this, but she was totally left out of all decision making by her husband and his doctor. After he died she was very upset and very angry. She felt she should have been involved in some way. All right, what is the obligation of the doctor towards her? They also had adolescent kids. The husband said, "Inform no one, I don't want them involved in this at all." Is there an obligation? I don't know.

Nagy: This is such a fundamental issue, and I think there will be a forcible change one day. Already a very brutal form of this issue is the

California case when the patient threatens to kill someone and the therapist, out of obligation to confidentiality, has a conflict that here is that person's life and here is my contract for the ethics of confidentiality of my contract with the patient. Yet, I think he is contracting ethically with the prospective victim because he may have the key of the victim's life in his hand. So he may say this is ridiculous, because all I am doing is treating a crazy patient, so I really had nothing to do with someone who is a lover or a neighbor of the patient, and yet, at that moment, when his patient might kill that person, he will be made contractually connected with the prospective victim.

I think that family members continually are prospective victims of any intervention on any one member. So I think that this is a fundamental principle which I think can only be solved by acknowledging that it exists! Well, some therapists are not capable or trained to live up to the contract. It doesn't remove the ethical implication of the contract. But actually, in treating any member of the family, I am in an ethical relationship, automatically, with all other members of the family, whether I see them or not, because their lives might be drastically affected by my work.

PART THREE

Anderson: As a background to a discussion of the ethics of intervention, I would like to recapitulate very briefly some of the contrast in the historical background both of medical ethics and of medical intervention.   I said there were two extreme examples: one is the traditional surgeon, who evolved from the barber, who performs primarily a technical job--and I used the example of lancing boils, which has now advanced to very complicated surgical procedures.   However these are procedures which are not seen as involving ethical issues, and they don't seem to involve value-systems in the minds of the people performing them.   A very skilled surgeon is like a very skilled computer programmer who knows how to do the job set before him.   He is not particularly concerned with the implications of what he is doing, or its impact on society, the family and so forth.

The other extreme from the surgeon-barber is the shaman-priest who is intensely involved in the social structure including the family, who derives his power not from the technique but from the participation of other people--the family, members of the tribe, from the society or group. His power depends almost entirely on this involvement and participation, whereas the barber-surgeon does not need this involvement--he can operate on a non-believer as well as on a believer.   This is not possible with a priest.

In the early days, in a stable society, where there were stable families, the operation of the technician didn't present many problems. The family could make the ethical or value-judgements about whether the surgical procedure should be done or not--they were willing to assume, and did assume, the responsibility for participation-judgement, which was kept within the family and out of the hands of the technician. Now a lot of the technology such as heart transplant or renal dialysis has many implications and consequences and affects value-systems throughout, not only in the family, but also society as a whole. The role of the priest-shaman has also continued to expand because, although we are no longer true believers in things other than technology, there is a continual under-lying involvement of very profound substance. We cannot escape our emotional involvement or commitments, we cannot approach a lot of problems in life without support--emotional and value--systems; so we have a need and we constantly demand that other people fulfill this shaman role.

An intact family in an intact society assumes a role in decisions. One of the reasons, I think, why there is an increase of ethical problems with the technology of medicine isn't that the technology has just increased so much, but the society and the family has just retreated from participation in making value-judgements and decisions.

I will now call on Ruth Cooperstock, who will talk about some problems connected with one technology used in medical care.

Cooperstock: Following yesterday afternoon, Henry very kindly had xeroxed a number of copies of an article by Albert Jonsen (who we all had hoped would be with us). Having read the article, I am now particularly sad that he is not with us, because I felt he directed himself beautifully to the issues that we are trying to deal with and that seem especially relevant. He pulled together many of the ideas that we are talking about--the special problems of technology and dehumanization. His entire concep-tual framework, his starting point, was so provocative that, for those of

you who haven't read it, I would suggest you do. He sees medical ethics
as dealing with three basic concepts and they are what he terms "the theory
of virtues" (in which one asks the question, What sort of person can rightly
be called a moral man?); "the theory of action," (in which one asks the
question, What ought I to do in this situation?); and the "theory of common
good" (in which one asks, What is the best form of human society?). And he
points out that it is the theory of common good that has been most ignored
in medical ethics; and then he expands on this in ways that I hope all of
us can discuss.

It seems to me that the profession has reached the point, not only
because of their technological development, but for a variety of reasons
involving the selection process into the profession and the current nature
of medical education where the idea of the common good has now been left
lying in the hands of the profession--almost unwittingly it has fallen
there, and the profession unknowingly has accepted a responsibility for
what they perceive to be the common good. I say "unknowingly," and I
think that is critical and very important. One is taught in medical
education that it is better to act than not to act; one has to intervene.
It is discomfitting to the actor not to act in situations in which someone
comes for help. One is taught, and one is socialized to believe, that it
is right and reasonable that the helping agent should tell the
client-patient what is correct therapy--"I know what is good for you and
therefore you should do it. Since you lack this expertise, you shouldn't
question my knowledge of this." It comes back to issues that Suzanne was
talking about yesterday, of knowing what is correct for, and imposing a

technology on people. Finally, it gets turned around so that the professional says, "I am doing this for your good anyway, so of course you must do as I say."

The special case I want to talk about is the case of chemotherapy, and particularly drugs which alter one's consciousness. Here, I think, what is interesting is that physicians fall into the role not of technologist but of shaman. The whole notion of the need for these drugs has arisen from the idea of people suffering from anxiety, from conditions that aren't readily measurable, that can't generally be seen and are totally subjective. These are drugs which are dispensed by general practitioners typically, and not by psychiatrists or other kinds of specialists.

Jonsen points out that it is the concept of the common good, the effect of medical technology on others, on society, on social institutions, that has been the most ignored aspect. And this is what is relevant to chemotherapy. A couple of years ago a group of us--Henry and myself and a group of others--held a Symposium. It was the first time, that I know of, that we dealt with some of the social aspects of the use of psychoactive drugs.

We are dealing with drugs which, first of all, are the most used drugs in the world, as a class of drugs. In North America, up to ten percent of the adult population will be swallowing one of these drugs on any given day. This is hardly a deviant case we are talking about; it is a large segment of the society we are talking about. We must also consider the expansion of the drug effects into their families, their work settings, into all the institutions in the society that they come into contact with. What is most significant, with the proliferation of these drugs, is that researchers have studied their effects on REM sleep patterns, on eye movement, on many aspects of one's physical state, and nobody has looked at the meaning to the individual who is using them in their everyday-life situation. The social toxicity, as Henry has so beautifully put it, has never been examined--such as the social-behavioural familial consequences of use. This is what we wanted to examine in terms of how do people perceive their world once they have used and are using psychoactive drugs. And I think these are two separate questions, as we have discovered, because people who are using drugs perceive their world somewhat differently, or are less able to talk about their perceptions of their world, than people who have used and are no longer using drugs.

Let me very briefly describe this research project that we have done. Then I want to read you a little of a transcription which, I think, in rather remarkable ways illustrates so many things that Harley has talked about, that Ivan and others here have talked about in general terms.

We invited volunteers who were using or had ever used minor tranquilizers, who would like to come in groups and discuss some of the social consequences of their use. We were absolutely overwhelmed with volunteers. We organized the groups, based only on their time convenience, and they met for two-hour periods. The groups, fourteen in all, ranged in size from five to eight people, with one accidental two-person group. Henry and I sat in on all sessions, and we tape-recorded the discussions. We opened each discussion by telling them the sort of thing we were interested in--the social consequences of drug use, and so on. Then we suggested that one person start by giving his or her history of tranquilizer use. We encouraged them to talk informally, ask questions of each other. They were sitting in comfortable chairs and had coffee available. The groups became very informal and comfortable very quickly. The first question that was frequently asked was, "Are you medical doctors?" Fortunately we were able to say no, because very clearly it would have altered the communication that took place.

The people who came were articulate, most were middle-class and had a high school or better level of education; they were people who had had both good and terrible experiences with drugs, and the range was over-whelming. I'm not going to talk about the physical consequences of use, which came up very commonly, and the sense of depression, and the lack of preparation for the drugs' effects and all the things which many of you are aware of. Certainly we learned an enormous amount about problems of addiction; we had people describe to us feelings of being a junkie, feelings of physical addiction to very tiny quantities, and so forth. But this isn't what is important today.

One respondent, a clergyman, had been taking these drugs for a number of years and he was very concerned with his use of them, and there was a great deal of self-loathing that he was able to articulate. He said, "I loathe myself for needing these drugs because they make me feel way deep down inside the way I've always wanted to feel all my life without ever taking anything." His whole sense of self was now built on the feelings that drugs gave him, and that without them the tensions, the pressures, the palpitations would return.

A psychologist said, "The first time I was given them, my first reaction to use of Valium. . . . I sort of felt, "Gee, if you had enough of this, somebody could tell you that your mother had died and you would say, 'Gee, that's nice.'" He said that feeling wore off, but that was his first reaction. Many people described this kind of feeling.

A large number of the people that we saw had been given these drugs, not because they had asked for them for some psychological illnesses, but in reaction to physical complaints. They either went to their doctor with chronic illnesses or a wide range of other somatic symptoms. There was a woman who had had a mastectomy, aged 25, and she was given them following it, and she had become totally dependent on them over a period of time. People with many kinds of chronic physical conditions were given these drugs: hypertension, back injuries, etc. Often they had been prescribed as muscle relaxants.

The tape transcription that I'm going to read from was of a woman who suffered from lupus. She was a most remarkable human being and I am terribly sorry I don't have the tape here because listening to it would give you a better sense of her and her experience than my reading bits from the transcript. She is, she explained, a bit of a medical freak in that she should have been dead years before; she had had this disease for almost fourteen years, and most people die of it in less time than that. She was currently in the process of forming a self-help group of lupus patients. Needless to say, she had had years of hospitalization. This extract starts when she first took ill and her first very severe attack. She had been put on antidepressants, tranquilizers and sleeping medication, all simultaneously. She says, "I finally got fed up with the whole scene. The psychiatrist with whom I was working kept insisting that I accept the fact that I was going to die." At this time her mother also had lupus. "And especially after my mother died, he said, 'Now will you accept that you are going to?' and I said, 'Go to hell.' I am alive and I am going to live. That's not the point. My husband and my daughter and I checked out of the country and went touring in Texas, and I came back determined that that was exactly what I was going to do. I went cold turkey off the Serax, the Valium and the Seconals, and I went through severe drug withdrawal. It was hell. I improved fantastically. I went into total remission. My cortisone finally was lowered. . . . I still have difficulty speaking because of the lupus, because of the arthritis, and I am still on fairly high doses of cortisone, and there is some brain damage that has taken place."

So that is the background. She says, "I have gone through drug with-drawal several times." She goes through severe drug withdrawal every time she gets her cortisone altered, as well as whenever she gets Valium or other medications. She says, basically there are two reactions. There is a physical reaction, "and that's not so bad" (that's with cortisone); "but there's a personality reaction that I go through. Usually I am very mild mannered, very happy-go-lucky. When I go through drug withdrawal, I can be fine one minute and literally blow my cool, or be an unadulterated bitch the next minute without any just cause. Or the slightest thing might trigger me, which is not my normal thing. I blow my cool maybe once a year and I find when I go through this, I blow it much more often. Or I go into very strong highs and lows." This is something that many people describe, in fact, when they lower their dosage--tremendous mood swings.

She said, "So again, this is part of my personality, this is part of my make-up. I just hate being sedated under any circumstances." We asked her, "Have you talked to other patients about these kinds of feelings?" She said, "Not so much. I've talked a lot to the doctors, and I've debated with them about it, but less with the patients. Some of them are quite content to be this way, they enjoy using crutches. You'd be amazed at the number of people who enjoy having a crutch, and the excuse for having a crutch. . . ."

She says, "I want to go back to where I said they were using drugs to cover up my feelings, because with as much anger and hate as I had in me, I never voiced my anger to my husband or to his family or to anyone at whom it was obviously directed. And they knew I was upset, as I was with just cause. So they gave me the Valium and the Serax and everything. But that didn't solve the problem at all because then they didn't know I was angry with them. Then one day I blurted it out and they came back and they grabbed me and they said, 'Why didn't you tell me? We kept doing this to you because you never said anything. You left yourself wide open.' Which was very true. You see, when you have lupus or any chronic disease. . ." (and I think this, too, is very relevant to things we have been talking about) ". . .many people tend to put you down. One beautiful statement they used to express to me was, 'You are so lucky to have your husband stick with you.' This is a constant one--'You are so lucky he

sticks with you.' Consequently you have to be better than normal. You
can't be the ordinary person who makes mistakes, who does things wrong.
You have to prove that you are superhuman, which is impossible. But you
keep trying, you see, because you make these demands upon yourself. And
when people make you angry you figure, 'Oh, I'm so lucky that you are
still sticking with me.' You are down about this low at this point, you
don't criticize. Even if they are out of line you don't put them down or
tell them off, because you feel that you are lucky. You are indoctrinated
to feel that you are lucky to have their friendship, you are lucky to have
this relationship, since because you are sick you shouldn't have anything,
you don't deserve anything. 'Poor kid, but we don't want to cope with
this.' Consequently, and I'm not alone in feeling this, we keep our true
feelings submerged. But the anger is there, the hurt is there, and until
you voice this hurt, until you listen to yourself, until you tell someone
when they are stepping out of line, it is never going to be corrected. I
keep going back--using Valium or Serax or any of these things to hide them
or mask them isn't going to solve any problems at all."

I'll stop now. I hope I haven't talked too long, but I think a lot
has been said here which deals with humanization and dehumanization.

Lennard: Thank you, for presenting this moving account. You brought
the personal experience of this woman right into this room!

Shands: One of the things that I hear is a kind of scapegoating of the
medical profession. It would seem to me that it's a good idea to put
this really into focus. I think that when one says that people are given
entirely too many drugs these days, it is absolutely true. We are all

inclined to be forced into that position, but I think it is easy to underestimate the degree to which that forcing is taking place. Particularly in New York City and New York State at the moment, the pressure against any kind of humanized service-delivery is enormous and is getting greater and greater. The evaluators and the accountability experts, and so forth and so forth, are continually forcing physicians, and other deliverers of health care, to document everything that they are doing, and to document tender loving care in thirty-minute sessions with a patient is a lot harder to do. It's a lot harder than the giving of some kind of drug is. We are paid the same amount for a clinic visit in which we write one prescription as we are paid for a clinic visit in which one allows the ventilation of anger, or sharing of other experiences.

Springer: There is one point that everybody started to lose sight of. I work in addiction research too. I think we have to blame the doctors, because they can prescribe drugs. They are prescribing substances which they know are acting on the brain, and they should know they are very superficially investigated. We know very little about the mental toxicity of these drugs. Due to the very important work of Dinkenberg and Felix Kreus we know very much more about cannabis than about any of the drugs that a lot of people are taking on prescription. And so I would blame the doctors for doing something they don't reflect about, knowing that they give substances acting on the brain, and believing the industry that such a substance is really an anti-anxiety drug, and not also a drug that harms some regions of the brain they don't know about.

Shands: It seems to me you are missing the point that, in the absence of prescription, drugs are freely available, and consumed in enormous quantities; tobacco or alcohol. Is alcoholism a disease?

Lennard: I think you know what Tom Szasz would say were he here--that the two issues are totally different. For example, if someone here wanted to jump off a bridge, I would say, "Please don't do it," and I would be very sad about it if they persisted, but ultimately it is their choice! If someone wishes to consume alcohol because he cannot bear the brutality of life, and that's how he chooses to kill himself, that's one kind of issue. Or if climbers go up the Matterhorn and fall off--which people do every day--that may be foolish but that is their decision, especially if they are experienced mountain climbers.

But for me, to do something damaging to others, in the name of therapy, is a totally different matter. These two issues therefore are not related. They often are confused in discussions.

Seeley: I think the argument is still badly framed. It appears to be now an argument as to whether the physician is altogether to blame, or wholly blameless, and either position is ridiculous. The physician cannot be scapegoated alone for partly being mystified and taken in by the absurd notion that mastery is everything and that, when the patient comes to him and says, "I have bad feelings or bad impulses," (whatever that may mean), "I want to master these," that he already, just as a person living in a civilization, shares that insane view of himself, and then contributes to his patient's mystification, and really, more in the guise of technologist than of shaman, gives him a little device for doing it. I don't think that

he can be held wholly exempt for being passively drawn into that.
Certainly the profession can't, particularly when one realizes that taking
that view also gives one manifest social and power advantages which otherwise one wouldn't have. So medicine is almost _the_ profession with which
all other professions compare themselves. On the other hand I agree that
until enough of us everywhere in the culture, whether it's in schools,
whether it's as parents, or whether indeed it is as persons (because most
of us have not learned that renunciation for ourselves), recognize that
the quest of mastery which is the core of this culture, ending up with the
absurdity of "I want to master my own feelings" and not even knowing what
the "I" is, what the subject of the sentence is, and the "me" that is the
object of the sentence--"I want to master me"--which is itself an extension of the word "self-control". . . . Until we learn to do that
culturally, until we alter all the other institutions, not a great deal
can be done!

But I do want to point out that at the very point when there was a
minor breakthrough, with all the risks and with all the follies--that is,
in the illicit drug enterprises of the early sixties, when people were
trying to use chemical substances to get out of this posture of self-
mastery and to permit the subordinated self to emerge into consciousness,
so that there were new awarenesses, new choices, however badly that was
managed, physicians and all the control apparatus--the police apparatus
of the society--moved as swiftly as possible to cut that off. There was
even a moment when people who were into pot in any serious way began to
hold tobacco, alcohol and the amphetamines and barbiturates in such con-
tempt that they would not use them. This had almost become a religious

truth, because these things cut you off from the feelings and the social
relations that pot, as they were using it, in a semi-ritual form, permitted
at least to some extent. And how did society react to these long-haired
people? It reacted with appropriate panic because, if that view had
succeeded, then the very nature of society would have been undermined.
How could you include such people as future executives? How would you
recruit them to be industrial workers? They wouldn't have that mind-set
anymore. So every endeavor was used to push that down, and to permit only
the State licensees to prescribe mind-altering substances. None of us was
innocent in that.

Shands: Are you saying that a personally selected mind-altering substance
is quite different from a professionally prescribed drug? It seems to me
that the mind-alteration by toxic substance is really common to both those
situations.

Seeley: Something altogether different was at stake. You went to a
physician and he gave you a drug that would enable you, or you and him
together, to do something in the name of some narrow aim: how to
"function in the world" (which usually means how to make a living in an
approved way). The kids I am talking about wanted to find out how to
surrender, because of their previous narrowing and training--wanted a
way to surrender to something that they sensed existed and that they sometimes found. I am not saying that it is the ideal way, but it was a wholly
different pursuit. And when they tried to talk to each other they were
unable to understand each other because all that the technologists, the
State-licensee-physician could think about, was how this affected whatever

it was that was being controlled. And what the others were asking about
was how to escape from that whole system, that whole way of looking at
life--no matter how clumsily they did it, and some of it wasn't altogether
clumsy.

Cooperstock: Could I say something about this? I really wanted to make
the point that these drugs are not just for mastery of the individual,
they are for masking and controlling. Large numbers of these drugs are
used to facilitate situations, social and familial, and you omitted this
from your discussion. I think this is terribly important. They are used,
for example, to keep women sedated whose husbands are alcoholics--so that
they won't be so upset by their husband's beatings, or their husband's
tossing their kids against the wall. And they are used in a multiplicity
of situations, particularly with women, to control their behavior. From
this point of view (and the medical profession goes along in this sense)
they are instruments of social control.

Shands: What I am really trying to say is, as I hear you, I think you
are really talking about symptoms.

Cooperstock: I am not talking about a symptom; I am talking about a
society.

Shands: Well, but I think the drug use in this society, voluntary or
professional, is more a symptom of a tremendous disorganization in the
whole society. And I think that we lose sight of the underlying disorganization, we lose track of how to try to understand that by
concentrating on a particular symptom, which seems to be exactly what the

physician does when he prescribes Valium to someone to avoid the awareness of the potential anxiety that the person has.

Lennard: This is a significant insight that I don't want to lose sight of.

Springer: One thing that I think is paradoxical is this mastery. Because if you read the ideology of illicit drug use, there also is an ideology of mastery in it. If you read Timothy Leary, what does he want to do--drive out emotions with LSD. If you read Ken Kesey he will try control by means of LSD. If you speak with heroin addicts the mastery afforded by the drug is one of the central goals. That mastery ideology, I think, is also in this area.

Seeley: It's part of it. To a very much lesser degree heroin--but certainly marijuana, hashish, peyote--were being used to escape into a different space. There was a surrender.

Lennard: It was also "better living through chemistry," though it may be living of a different sort through chemistry. There is no doubt that there was a difference in the kinds of emotions that people wanted to experience and that intimacy and closeness were important to the "counter-culture"--so that there may be differences in the kinds of experiences aimed for. Rather than doing well on the job and taking Valium so that one shouldn't appear disorganized, by taking pot one wanted to be able to be intimate with others and relate to them!

Seeley: We are talking about a polarity that does go to the center of all these questions. There was a sufficient group for whom this was a means for surrender and not mastery--which is a crucial question for our society. We have forgotten the arts of surrender--surrender to ourselves or others.

Anderson: Are you saying some drugs were used for the art of mastery rather than other techniques, and that drugs are even used for the art of surrender?

Seeley: I think that most of the prescribed drugs are used to permit the ego to dominate every other aspect of the personality, by and large--or for social control, but that at least for a very short time before it was stamped out, many of the soft, psychotropic drugs were very much more similar in their use to the way the Indians used peyote--to enable them to escape into an enlarged inner space and an enlarged outer space which had a different relation to the cosmos and to the reflection of the cosmos within. That's a very different employment, for the object is to let the ego abandon that control, and to give up and to let happen.

Lennard: Maybe we can put the issue into the terms of this morning's topic: What are the ethics of intervening in this manner in the lives of these patients? And I would like us to keep in mind the responsibility of the intervenor, not only to those to whom he directs his interventions, but to all those who are affected by that intervention.

Shands: What I would suggest is that we also broaden it to include regulators of the intervenors. Because there are many places where we have very little choice these days.

Anderson: All right, now can we get to the Nagy talk? Perhaps Ivan can say some things about his discussion of yesterday afternoon and bridge it to the top of this morning. Particularly, I would like to see him relate issues of accountability to the patient-therapist role.

Nagy: Let me try it in a certain way. I would like again to sharpen some of the premises, and then I would like to talk, strategically, from two separate points of view. The premises, again, are ethics-as-a-dynamics-of-a-relationship. I am not talking about what this or that history of ethics book says. It is not value-ethics. It's not the listing of value-priorities. It's not: Who is the morally good man? Who is the bad man? I know families in which there is this kind of format of thinking. I remember a Dutch family I interviewed a couple of months ago in Holland. The father was a good man; the mother was a good woman; but only that father could never talk to any of the seventeen children when, on his birthday, they got together. Could he talk with his wife? No! They couldn't talk with each other. But it was a "good marriage!" So this would be an example, maybe, of value ethics; that a person has to be good or bad, and that it is inside of the person-- goodness and badness. This is not the kind of ethics I am talking about. Nor is it the other phrase we heard this morning: "the common good." Now that has some ethical implications. Common good is something that is good for all of us. Like what the utilitarian philosophers talked about: that we are all peers and that if all of us are good and the society will do good for all of us, then all of us will be happy and that it is morally good to have such a society. To me, both these notions lack what I would

call a dialectical characteristic. Someone is good, this one's bad;
grandmother was good, grandfather, bad. This is a non-dialectical world
in which there are these finite ultimate judgements about whole persons
that they are either good or bad. To me there is a third interesting
ethics which I call a dialectic of relational balances, in which there is
a constant fluctuation of I and you in the relationship with me. And,
therefore, there is a balance of interests, balance of survivals, balance
of satisfactions, balance of fairness. That is a dynamic which is being
lived from minute to minute. So as a therapist, also, I am not saying
what is good. I am, however, actively influencing people to work on their
balance. So I am not going to tell that you are selfish, and you are
being exploited. I am saying, "Well, why don't the two of you look at
this?" I mean: He sounds like he is saying that you are being selfish.
What about it? So at that point I really make them look at their own
balance. It is really only these two who live it, not an outsider, that
can determine what the balance is. To me it may look like, that if she
says he can never have any drinks at home, that maybe this is unfair. Or
if he says that she couldn't ever do this and this. But for them, maybe
this is not a major item. So only they can see what balance is what. We
heard also another version: anger at mother for bringing her into the
world. Well, again, what is the item here about accountability? It this
statement made by the child who is saying, "My parents, by bringing me
into the world, should have been accountable for doing at least the average
minimum things for me that would secure that my life would be a satisfying
one. And since, somehow, I feel thay have not done that, they have not
lived up to this accountability. Therefore, I am angry for having been

brought into this world." So here is the psychology of being angry at
the parent, transformed into an ethical language of balances, of what one
is accountable to, and what one is entitled to get, as a result of the
other one's accountability, and I feel the balance is off. So I can
resent my parents because the balance is off.

These are some of the premises of the ethical dynamic. We can go
from here to societal understanding or go into therapeutic understanding.

I will try to connect with the issues we were just talking about.
And here I think Harley's comment helped me, when he asked, "Are we
talking about symptoms, or are we talking about some kind of underlying
social disintegration which has many other aspects, including the bureau-
cracies of government organization, and so on?

To me, as a strategist, I differentiate between two levels, depending
again on the ethical impact of lives or interactions. I can look at life
(as Henry talked about, or Tom Szasz would have said here) the dignity of
the individual who should be allowed to be autonomous and free, and if he
wants to kill himself it is his business and he should have that freedom
if he really makes that decision. This is somewhat similar to me to the
utilitarian ethics, in which there are parallel individuals only--there
are citizens A, B, C, D, who are roughly equals in potential consequence
to each other; one is maybe a little stronger or older, but basically they
are interchangeable citizens, and something goes on between them which is
either good or bad. I felt that many of our comments this morning were
on this level, that we could do better about this or that symptom of what
happens in society.

In contrast to this, to me, the intergenerational differential that exists between a parent and a child is a discontinuous realm. There you cannot talk about these things. "Here is my little newborn child, and my philosophy is to let him do what he wants and decide for himself. I am not going to intrude, I respect his integrity and freedom. If he decides to jump off the window it is his decision. . . ." Obviously it doesn't work in the intergenerational context! There is an inevitable intrusion--you can call it enabling, you can call it generative, you can call it procreative, parenting, guiding, forming, educating. This is very different from any notion of democratic or liberalistic regard where you have just as much freedom as I have. This is a different realm.

I think the strategy really lies here. I think what happens to society is in this realm, where the new generation is being messed up right from the beginning, irreversibly, with a degree of impact which is several orders of magnitude higher than what takes place between a drunken adult and his doctor, or a drug-addicted adult and a bureaucrat. Well, something might be changed there too; that drunk could drink a little less, maybe, or drink it in a more constructive way. But this is not comparable in terms of strategic importance to the level in which now a new generation is being developed from, let's say pregnancy on--the interuterine damage to the brain, the early experiences, and so on.

I don't know yet what to do with it, but I feel that we can go in both directions and I would like to. . . . In my mind, as a family therapist, in my experience as a therapist, as a human intervenor, the exciting

and important thing lies in that second dimension--in the intergenerational. Much much less happens in the peer relation between adults, which
is very important, because adults have more power. In no-fault divorce
it really affects the freedom of adults, yes; but what happens to the
children in the meantime, who just then grow up irreversibly this way or
that way? That to me is a much more exciting issue, as a strategic or
therapeutic agent.

So again when we talk here about these matters I would say that what
happens with the adults is more on the symptom level--that's the way it
looks when life is messed up. Whereas the level of the children is maybe
where we can prevent life from being messed up. What are those strategies, what can we do about it? What can we do about those masses of
people who are out there--girls who get pregnant at fourteen, and no one
cares.

Lennard: It is fascinating, and interesting, that you feel that you
don't have a value position. Your position is that we should be more
concerned about intergenerational issues. It is a value position! And
then one could counter that by saying, "What happens to those kids we
are concerned about is, of course, ultimately affected by what we do to
their parents. So that a mother who is given phenothiazines may, in my
view, become a poorer mother; or a person with a long-term illness, such
as cardiac disease who is not permitted to deal with this illness in his
family context may damage the development of a young child. Your view
is a system view, that you see how these systems impinge on each other
and have an impact on each other. But it is also a value position.

Nagy: Henry, what I'm saying is that my value statement is that it is more important to take care of how the hydrogen bombs are guarded than to take care of how the old-fashioned gunpowder supply is guarded. You can say that this is a value position. But I think that it is also a reality. The hydrogen bomb is more important to control than the old-fashioned gunpowder.

Bloch: Can I just jump in with one other thought about this: Ivan's position is a tactically much more powerful position. It is a position on which we have a chance to do something. If there is any rallying point around which human beings, no matter where they come from, no matter how crooked and corrupt and evil they are, can genuinely be rallied, it is just on this score of how children are treated and what happens in a family. It is true that children have been, through history, mistreated beyond words. But the phenothiazine question can, in terms of the effect on the prenatal development of the child, be made vivid. It is a tactically powerful point because the intuitive human understanding of this is enormous. If there is any place where people can be agreed, it is around being good to children. That doesn't mean that they are always good to children--we can be terrible to children; we can malnourish them; we can do all kinds of things. But, at least, given the range of operating possibilities, it is a tactically powerful position. You can get mothers to stop smoking during their pregnancy when you can't get people to stop smoking at any other time. You can get them to stop taking drugs, to eat well during their pregnancy.

So I want to say this has a tactical value in addition to its strategic value.

Seeley: I tire of sounding monotonic, but I am appalled. Perhaps, in a sense even more by Don's comment on the view than the view itself, though I think it is a proper inference from the view. To me it is inconceivable that well-parented children, beloved, treated as best we know how, with all the entitlements granted, so that they immediately feel satisfied, growing up in a scheme where they gladly assume the responsibilities, because of the satisfaction of the entitlements--it is an appalling thought that anyone can believe that that will, when they walk out of that room into the other institutions, enable them to decide when or whether to press the button, how to manage vicarious relations between China and Russia, so that we will not be involved either in a two-cornered or three-cornered war; or how to, or whether to, so reduce the level of technology and standard of living so that indeed the rest of the world will be able to live, that there won't be a dying third world which we either have to deaden our conscience to while we watch it die, or turn our guns against it so it won't invade us. That those things will be solved by those means--NO. I have lived my whole life in caring for the things that you care about. But to say that that is the tactical, the strategic point--even neglecting the time aspect--that by the time three generations have gone by to allow that to really happen, that we can turn our attention there, and not here, and not attend to that school in which that child will be put, which will undo whatever good work is being done. . .

<u>Bloch</u>: That is an exaggeration which you know is not a position which I would hold. We have to move on all of those fronts, and I don't have a kind of brainless indulgence of just feeding a child endlessly and it will grow up to be a happy, decent, humane individual. However, I do see occasionally a little glimmer of hope in the world, and I would like to cite the very group that you were talking about, who were trying to use, let us say, chemicals, in a way to free themselves. Most of them were kids from the families who had made this kind of an ethical commitment to their children. I see them among my grown children, who are different but who are pleasing and ethically responsible and are trying to live in different ways in the world, to be givers rather than takers, to not be consumer oriented. And I see my own children, in some sense, being better than I was.

<u>Anderson</u>: A lot of what Ivan said this morning seems to be a feeling about using the issues of values within the family system. And this seems to be also what Henry, and to some extent John, have expressed: that these same principles should apply also to being professional furnishers of health care. That to some degree the physician in prescribing drugs is acting <u>in loco parentis</u>, and should have some of the same dynamics, or the interchange which is described by Ivan as between parent and child. In a way, we are giving to the furnisher of health care this role, and we have the expectation of him, the responsibility. I think Henry is thinking of a dialectic in this area. Am I correct, Henry?

<u>Lennard</u>: I think it is a very interesting parallel, and I do wish to stress what is the responsibility of the physician in this area. I don't

think we can escape the issue by simply saying there are many ways of working and there are many ways of conceiving of oneself in the doctor or therapist role. Yesterday we discussed something that was rather subtle--What is the responsibility of the analyst? Is it his responsibility to point out to his new patient that during the analysis there may be turmoil in the family, that the children or parent of the analysand may get upset due to the vicissitudes of the interaction of analyst and patient? Is there a need for a physician, or a therapist to consider these outcomes which may or may not occur? Is there, in other words, something to be said about an "ethics" of intervention, about principles that govern what the therapist needs to inform the patient about? What is the responsibility of the chemotherapist who is giving treatment to one member of the family who may seriously disrupt and disorganize everybody's life, to at least inform other people about the possible outcomes of this intervention? To take into account the fragility and the integrity of the family in doing this? In some sense, Ivan did answer this; and he said yesterday, and I think should say today again for all of us, that he feels the intervenor needs to consider all others on whom his intervention has an impact. We need to consider the families of all who come in. These are issues that are not really talked about. Now why aren't they discussed? Al Johnson would have said, as a member of human experimentation committees, that some doctors have an underdeveloped sense of ethics. But it might be better if he said it than if I do. Maybe it's a professional characteristic, maybe not.

Nagy: I think some of the things, as I recall, that came up yesterday were a distinction which is very important, especially in the development of family therapy over the years. Here we are, not so much talking about imposing inappropriate therapeutic involvement on relatives. Could you tell this patient that they should bring their relatives? Or could you tell the relatives that they consider themselves as patients also? For these actions, all of us have had different degrees of reluctance, though some early family therapists inversely had a mission for doing them. But, on the other hand, there is another issue there, which is different from seeing everybody together in that room and making them come and talk in front of each other, sharing the patient's role and all this kind of stuff that early family therapy was very enthusiastic about.

The issue I am raising is--whether you call it family or any kind of therapy, any kind of human intervention--whether you acknowledge it or not, your intervention will not be confined to one person. You say, "Well, I only see this one so my work is confined only to this one." In physical medicine that is possible, maybe, but even there it is not possible. But, at least, as a surgeon I know that I only cut one person, and I don't cut the brother and the sister physically. But obviously in psychotherapy anything I do to one person will inevitably and absolutely affect anyone who is in a relation with that person. I can take the position that I don't want to know that, that I am not interested in it. I am ethically not considering myself bound by this. But that does nothing to the ethical reality which is that I do intervene in the lives of those others.

I believe we must acknowledge this, and what I do is not only to acknowledge this but to offer my help. I am not saying you and you and you are all my patients and you have to come or else you will get terribly sick or something. But what I am saying is that although so-and-so is my patient I know that others may need my help, and I do find myself in an advantageous position to help all of them, since I know about them because they are members of the same family. So I offer that help to the grandfather, the grandmother, and so on. My recommendation is that we should think everything through from the point of view that includes the interests of all of these people. And if they can accept my help I am glad to offer my help to them. If they all come, it is even better. This way, even if you see only one person from the beginning to the end, you consider what happens to the others. If you do this and this, what will it do to your marriage? What will it do to your mother? Or your child, or whatever? Or else, let's ask your mother, let's ask your wife--you ask your wife or your mother. Or maybe you bring him or her in here. These are variations--and they may look like a conjoint session. They may look like an individual session, or they may be my asking an individual to go and talk to his relatives and report what happened. All these things are technical details. The main thing is that, ethically, the contract should be, and is, with all of those whose lives are being affected by the intervention. This can't be denied or ignored.

Lennard: This is a very fundamental point, which often is not understood. As interventions get more and more potent, and as the interventions affect more and more, everybody is involved with the persons who are the targets of interventions. This point should be emphasized, thought about, and spelled out in considerable detail--it is a matter of good medicine to involve the family of a diabetic in getting information about the disease, and what the interventions mean to the family. It may even be unethical not to spell out for them what the interventions may do to the everyday life of the family. It is both a technical problem which is being ignored, and an ethical problem, which is not being thought about. It is bad medicine and bad ethics to ignore it.

Bloch: I would like to dilate on that just a little bit, quickly. Along the line of what is practical, the physician knows what he can afford to know, just like all of us. Part of what is missing, I think, along lines that have been indicated here this morning is: What is the condition of this person? We are mostly talking about people who if they allowed themselves in the course of any day to know what came through their office, they would go psychotic by the end of the day. Because, if you take a general practitioner's office, and you watch the forty or fifty people in pain, misery, malfunction, economic difficulty, itching, sleeplessness, vomiting, diarrhea. . .and just simply allow yourself to experience that as a living fact, it is impossible. There is no way it can be experienced without going crazy. And I am talking about the physician who graduated from an adequate medical school in the middle of his class, a decent guy who reads the journals--he can't stand to know what he could know, let alone to know what the effects of the drugs are, or what the family's lives are like, or even what his own family is like. Because every night he goes home exhausted, defeated, having failed to do most of everything

he set out to do, because most conditions can't be cured--at best they
can be ameliorated. And then he goes home to people who are hungry
psychologically, emotionally deprived, grabbing at him. And I have a
practice full of men like that: radiologists who are treating cancer
patients--they can't afford to know what the life of those cancer patients
is like, because if they did they would be psychotic. Now if we want to
talk seriously about the human events, this is, I think, the level we have
to approach. And it is idle to rail at those people. Sure, they are
inadequate--deliberately. They cannot survive if they are adequate. I
see three or four or maybe five families a day, in a spacious office,
comfortably. I have all kinds of protection. I can afford to know
certain things, simply because I am enormously protected. My self-esteem
is protected. I am not made to feel helpless and defeated.

Now, surely, that's only a piece of it again. I realize that the
drug-industry complex is enormously powerful, and feeding on that misery,
and offering some ways in which people can be helped temporarily to ease
that pain. But that is the sea of human misery, that flows through any
doctor's office every day of the week. We don't pay enough attention to
that. We are not getting anywhere near this issue.

Kremser-Springer: I don't think that that is quite the point. Because,
if you take a patient who is chronically ill, for instance with diabetes,
or, what I am concerned with, gynecological diseases, such patients are
not only out-patients, they are sometimes in hospitals. And at this
point, for instance, the doctor in the hospital can easily afford half
an hour, or longer, during the day, to let the family, or the husband and

the children come and to talk with him about what "hypoglycemia" means, and what the family can do. This is not done. For instance, in the out-patient clinic where I am working, when the patients are examined, there are doctors who don't even talk a word with them. They have an assistant give them a prescription. But this is not a question of lack of time. And it is not a question of time in the private offices either. And this is not done.

Bloch: I think I know how that world in the hospital works. I think if we had time to build on this foundation of understanding of the human condition, and the selection of physicians--and who goes in, and how the whole organization is arranged--I agree, changes could be made. I don't think it is a hopeless matter. There is some room for movement. We have to take into account this piece of it, that's all.

Cooperstock: What you describe is perfectly true, and it is documented by all the statistics on doctors' longevity and on their alcoholism rate, their use of drugs, and even their suicide rate. We know this, of course. This is not an exoneration. The implication of what you said is that we have to expand our health-care-delivery-system, so that doctors don't see so many patients each day, so that there are more doctors, and so on. I don't think this is what you meant, but it is an implication.

I would like to return to other questions: Why are the people in those offices? Do they belong there? What other kinds of services need to be and can be provided? What do we see, as responsible persons, should be provided as alternatives--whether it be self-help, whether there are

other kinds of services, whatever they are? How can we de-medicalize?
This is the critical point to make.

Bloch: I agree with that. I think a really systematic systems analysis
of this would then say what pieces of it we can change. I see many that
we can change. I think, for example, I would like to see medical students
really having the kind of teaching that Ivan is talking about. I would
see that a medical student's attention to the systems situation in his
own family would be a critical point. He would recognize and be helped
early to understand that his tie to his own family is one of the most
significant features of the way he is going to practice medicine, and that
he must conserve those balances in some fashion so that he himself is
nourished and able to function. I think that the bringing in of other
professionals to pick up the pieces that he is not interested in and not
trained for can be very, very helpful. I think that there are ways of
de-medicalizing so that many of the people who come in the office can,
with genuine kindness and compassion, be dealt with by people who do not
have those special skills. There are many things that can be done.
However, it is essential to take this whole unit of the system, including
the physician, his family, his family of origin, and to include those in
some fashion as equally relevant with these other issues.

Nagy: I would like to tighten some of the points made. Maybe it would
be helpful. The question emerges here: Where does dehumanization start?
And maybe there are two major levels that we haven't yet connected. The
one is in the intra-familial realm of alienation; it is in the intergenerational, and as you suggested, in the isolation and disconnectedness

where there should be more meaningful connections in families. The other one would place itself somewhere on the peer-level interaction, systemic and organizational rules in society, and so on, which is in this much larger territory of societal organization.

I think that this is a very important issue, because somehow we have to relate the levels to each other. We seem to be talking at one time about one, and another time about another, as if we had solved the problem of their interaction.

Another issue comes up in philosophising about ethics: What is practical? I am practicing the position I expressed here every minute of my practice, from the first moment when I see a family. This ethical leverage is an enormous therapeutic strategic device. For instance, let's say my attitude to a pregnant woman who takes drugs is that I would like to help her take less drugs. I can approach her on the level of herself (let's say it's smoking): think of the possibility of cancer, what do you think of smoking that much? Or I can approach her from the point of view of her husband's irritation about her smoking; or I can say, "You are pregnant, and it may damage your child." This is an escalating ethical realm. The first one is ethically indifferent, as far as I am concerned. If you are smart, if you think about it, you don't want to end up with a miserable disease which ruins your life at an early age--that's not an ethical issue from my point of view, that's a question of smartness or discipline of living. The second one already has ethical implications-- that your husband is a nice guy and maybe you want to consider his interests, plus whatever you get back from the relationship. The third one is really a very sharply ethical issue: You are pregnant, your child might be affected irreversibly; now you can do something about it, later it will be too late; do you want to face the responsibility. And I think here is the highest degree, in my experience, of strategic intervention, whether a person is alcoholic or whatever, it is in this realm of sharpening the ethical dynamic. If you know how to utilize that, that is the highest leverage for therapeutic intervention. If you can sharpen the ethical implication you bring the highest pressure for change.

I am trying to connect now the "practical" and philosophical because I think we are not just talking here about descriptive neat categorization, but we are talking about the sharpest ethical issues, provided we know how to work this.

Lennard: I like that very much. It is a value position. I like it because it does get us away from the problem which I had posed when we met before and that has to do with the fact that often one person can get better at the expense of other people. Or other people are not growing sufficiently with that person and that person is able to do things but everyone else in the family is then worse off. Some family therapists will almost say proudly that when the son got better the father got a coronary, as if they were able to perform such magical things with their powerful interventions.

Your kind of modest definition of the liberation of relational resources says that you are not really doing anything if all the people in the situation aren't getting something out of it. I think that is very good. I don't think one can argue scientifically that this is a scientific position but it is a nice human position which I like.

Bloch: There has been so much reference to the noxious effect of the family, and then the denial of this, that we are not talking about an individual or a family but the situation. I think it is very important to emphasize how can you help the family understand and act, and thereby help the patient. And in the case cited, it might well require pointing that out to the family: that although they might feel that the individual is being made to suffer unnecessarily and would be better off finally dead, the patient herself may not feel that way; and the family may have to be helped to understand that, for better or worse, that patient wants to live, in that gruesome situation, and that they can help that situation by not putting still a further stress on that patient.

I think I prefer to pick up on the first part of the question that you raised, and that part has to do with training and the nature of trust.

The way that I think about this (and it's because of the colleagues that I work with) really has to do with trying to conceptualize the nature of the therapeutic encounter, and with trying to understand, first of all, who is involved in it. It is very evident in family therapy that there are people involved in it--or, if you want to put it in non-personal terms, there are systems involved in it. For example, a critical system is the gender system of the therapist. As a male therapist, I am in a significantly different system in relation to the people who come to me; and so

the therapeutic encounter is informed and colored by my sex. In dealing
with a family--let's take even a simple family, as a man and a woman and
perhaps one child--my relation to all those people is determined by whether
I am a parent, and by my sex. It is determined in the same way that other
encounters are.

In a more durable kind of way, the fact that I am an older brother or
a younger sister, the fact that I come from a particular cultural and
socio-economic group, all of those things influence what I do in a family.
My way of even conceiving of the problem, where I am in my own life, how
old I am, again influence and color and even create the very things that
I can see. What I can perceive is not simply a function of what is out
there, but it's a function of my interaction. And my interaction not just
as a person, but as a representative of a number of different complex
social systems that overlap.

How do I relate this to training? I think that, in a general way, one
moves through life, if one is fortunate, enlarging one's ability to see
and understand those factors that influence the shape of the therapeutic
encounter. And that changes. It has been changed for me by this meeting.
But there are some very durable and stable systems that are highly influ-
ential. I think there are qualities I have as a person and as a therapist
my sensitivity, my compassion, my ability to be trustworthy, which are all
somewhat present, but not ultimately, not completely so. I am somewhat
compassionate within the limits that the system permits me, the systems I
am a part of. And these are personal systems (as well as being systems
that affect all the society). We teach in a way that tries to help this

be a growing process for the people who work with us. And we have specific
ways to do that--it's not just a wish. For example, people who study with
us, among other things, study their own families. They try to change their
own families. They try to understand what their limits are, and modify
those in terms of the systems that they can actually influence, which are
the private individual networks that they are a part of.

I think I am indicating that this is an unending and continuous quest
for everybody, that it should go on until the moment we die. But somewhere,
the position one takes influences the shape of the therapeutic encounter.
One can see oneself as a technologist, as a manipulator of skills. And in
family therapy we have powerful tools--we have the tools of paradox, we
have the tools of negative injunction. We can produce very profound
effects. We have a struggle within that branch of the profession as to
where one is in relation to those powerful tools. My own feeling is that
they have to be used within the overall context of an awareness of oneself
in the therapeutic encounter. Let me just put that in as one building
block that seems at least to be useful. The way of looking at it permits,
perhaps, a better approximation to an answer to the kind of question we
are dealing with.

Shands: It is implied in what you said that there is something wrong with
the family that you come in contact with, that there is something that
should be changed. Is that right?

Bloch: It is implied that there is something wrong with me--I'll start with
that. It is implied, that is, that I am in some continual growth and
change. And, that there are options; and that some options are better than

other options. There is a way of proceeding that comes very close to education, as opposed to therapy. I think the nature of the therapeutic encounter says, as I see it, that this is an interactive decision. I liked the notion of our Viennese colleagues as they spoke about analysis-- that someone comes into the office and says, "I am homosexual." And you say, "Well, fine, but let's see what does that mean to you. You have come here for some reason, and let's together try to discover what it is." Now it may be that in the process of discovery something else will turn up. The person will say, "Really I feel very much out of touch with other people--I don't know how to get connected to other people." The problem changes in the course of the interaction. Now, that's an interactive definition that is a growing and changing one. For example, I use a notion of "linked contracts." I assume that someone comes into the office (or a family comes into the office) and they have something along that line So we work for a while, and we get somewhere, at which point I say, "Well, OK, do you want to re-negotiate another contract? Do you want to move some step forward?"

It happens that there are some people who want to continue in therapy, but I can't have them in my office because they bore me. They cease, in some fashion, to engage me. And, on occasion, I terminate treatment with people or with families (who want to continue working) because I am no longer engaged by them. So I make a decision on my side of the interaction And I think that is not so uncommon. I think it happens. I say, "I think we've gotten as much out of this as possible, there's nothing more that I can say that would be useful."

Nagy: A few comments in trying to put things together--because I fear the
break between the micro-cosmic and macro-cosmic levels. We talk about
family and family therapy, and then we talk about society. I was assigned
to have some concern about ethics or justice (by Henry I think)--which,
of course, I would have without his assigning me, anyway. And then we
were asking: Does something have to be wrong with every family?

This brings me to a number of questions. Are we here to talk about
our society? What is our society? We assume that we who work in New York
or Philadelphia and those who work in Vienna are talking about the same
society. Now, maybe to some degree there is similarity. I grew up in
Budapest which was closer to Vienna than New York. I think it is quite
different from New York and Philadelphia. Now, if we talk about India
and Guatamala and places like that--are we dealing with these issues, are
we covering those human territories? That is one of my questions because,
as we talk about justice and ethics, I would like to come back to my two
major aspects of an ethical dynamic of relationship. The one is "entitlement," and the other, the inverse of it: in my terms, "accountability."
I am either entitled, or, if I have already taken a lot, I am accountable.
If I am accountable, I either act on it and repay, or at least acknowledge
that I am taking, whereupon I begin to be indebted, or perhaps even guilty.
So it is a balance. Giving increases entitlement. Receiving increases
accountability. Doing wrong increases accountability. Doing good
increases entitlement. This is basic mathematics. It is very similar to
accounting of a financial type. And I think every ethics, every relational
ethics, is an accounting system--it's a quasi-methematical system.

I was wondering this morning why we went past so rapidly a very important question when we talked about the obligation on the part of society, the so-called "just society," or "society of the common good." There are the professions--which are an elite of trained people, people who make good incomes and so on. And then there are the masses of people who don't know as much or don't have as much money. They are being served, presumably, and they pay the taxes, and they should receive some benefits. So that there is an obligation to inform the consumer-masses of people, to treat them fairly, not to exploit them unfairly, and so on. And they are entitled to fair receiving.

Now, in my judgment, this is related to the idea of distributive justice: that there should be an equality between receiving and giving benefits. And I think that Western democracy has been in love with this idea. One labor union has the right to get just as much as, or even a little more than, the other union; and then the other union has the right to get just a little more than the first. Everyone has a right to get. "It's unfair, they get more"--this kind of thing. This is related to welfare ethics or to women's rights in some way, and to the whole issue of technology. Technology is a form of wealth, and the question is: How is it being distributed? Or sexuality, as Philip Rieff put it, is a major commodity of civilization. How is it distributed? A rich man--like King Farouk--he can have all his pornography (he apparently had a vast collection of pornography as well as good-looking women)--and the poor person can't have it; he has to be moral, whereas the rich need not. Bishops during the Renaissance could be "above" the morality of the average person. So these are also questions of the justice of distribution of goods. To me this is all the ethics of entitlement.

But when we talk, for instance, about another thing--let's say ecology, or overpopulation--then we talk about the ethics of accountability. We are saying, "It's not only: Does this person get more, and does another guy get more, and does another guy get more than you do, but: What are you responsible for?" I think that wealthy and successful societies somehow lure their populations into believing that they should get more. The wealthy administrators of society and the high aristocracy feel guilty that they have so much. So they want to make the people feel that *they* can also get more and more. So somehow the successful societies get trapped into emphasizing the ethics of entitlement--that you must just be sure that you get what you are entitled to. What are you accountable for? Well, you don't have to be accountable any more because we are so successful that we can give it to you. And, I think, this may kill the balance. The young people who have nothing but this lose an active relationship to life. This is passive: to sit there and see just what is flowing my way, without my being accountable for something. And I think, then, maybe I have to stimulate myself to get more, and even more, and even more. Maybe now I can get more only by taking drugs. So this way of thinking may help us understand the "drug problem."

One more point. One aspect of this which may undo all of what we are talking about very quickly is irresponsible parenting. This is where I think accountability fits the most, and I think this is where the weak point

of society lies. We can legislate fair distribution and fair use of technology and so on, but while we are doing so, some people throw millions of
children into society, out of a deep structural hostility, without caring
about those children, without caring about ecology. And those children are
of course entitled to be treated with full rights, but they will take away
from the others because of their surplus existence. Not only that, but
because they are not parented by their parents, they will take more welfare
And so on.

Somehow I think that the sense of accountability is missing in society
in the family, as well as on a large scale. It starts with producing
children irresponsibly, it starts with not taking care of children--and it
leads into the limitless welfare system, it leads into the children who are
entitled just to get because they were not given, and to a-further decay of
accountability. And, of course, down the drain goes the clean water, the
clean air, the food supplies, and reasonable distribution of the advantages
of society.

I would like to come back to emphasizing that the balance of entitlem
over accountability somehow has to be built into every human relationship,
microcosmic or macrocosmic. When we think about a broad philosophy of
improving things, we cannot just think of fairness of distribution (which
is entitlement ethics) but we have to connect it with how people are
accountable in return. Even the poor people. In fact, the poor people
may be the ones who violate accountability just as badly if they refuse to
be parents in a parenting-accountable sense, and become mass producing
parents in a merely biological sense.

<u>Sapir</u>: I want to cite a little project that makes a somewhat different point. This is a project for parent education in a pediatric well-baby clinic in Mount Sinai Hospital. We gave money for the pilot phase of this project. This was a simple idea to take advantage of the long periods of waiting when mothers are sitting with their babies or children in the waiting room. The hospital had already provided a little playroom for the children. Dr. Morris had the idea that it might be helpful and useful to take advantage of this situation to educate the parents, to teach them how better to interact with their children, how to play with them, how to read to them, how to use toys, and so on.

She did a little film strip on this program, and arranged, with our help, to have a new sound track done. And it is an excellent sound track which shows how well a competent film-maker can do. She was sensible and sensitive enough to have recorded some of the experiences of the mothers who had gone through this program, and a very simple message came out as you talked with these lower-class, disadvantaged, Black and Spanish American mothers. One mother said, "I have to confess this program really turned me off at first; I really resented it. But I have got to tell you that I have completely changed my mind. I didn't realize that I could educate my child. I didn't realize that a child needed the help of its mother to learn how to understand things, how to talk, how to read, how to play, how to solve simple puzzles." And another mother would say, "Look at me. I have educated my child for three years and it isn't even in school yet. I don't have to wait until it goes to school." Another mother said, "I just assumed that a child learned when it was ready, but I have learned that I can be a teacher." This was a big thing. These mothers did not realize that they were agents capable of and responsible for bringing up and educating their children. These people thought that they had to go to the expert, to the teacher. And evidently it was a very revealing and meaningful experience for them. It was certainly a revealing experience for me to hear them say this simply and directly.

I don't know how this fits into entitlement and accountability, and I don't want to sound pollyannaish, but an enormous amount can be done by simple education at the right time.

Bloch: I would like to build on that a little bit. One of my colleagues is working with people who work with cancer patients and their families. The families are enormously threatening to the professionals who work with the patients. The problem is that if the patient is entitled because of being either close to the end of his life or close to some serious disability, the family is then seen as being another group of people who come to the professional and say, "Give me." There are then four hungry mouths instead of one hungry mouth, psychologically. The notion that they can become a resource for each other rather than drain things into themselves from the outside world, that they can turn to each other and out of the strength and resources of the family itself that they can help with the healing or help with the work that needs to be done, is simply not even known to the professional yet. That is, the professionals don't even think of it in terms of restoring this natural healing balance. And this lack increases the panic of the professionals who feel drained and less able to relate in any kind of way, tend more and more to fragment, to specialize, to do more and more of the things that we have talked about. But I think

on this middle level--neither on the most microscopic nor the most
macroscopic social level--that there is a possibility of taking this kind
of orientation, and to act in these care situations and enhance the humanity
of everyone concerned, including the care-givers.

It seems to me possible, in a modest and limited way, with this kind of
an orientation, to make better and more constructive moves in some of the
situations we are concerned with.

Seeley: I am more and more troubled by this fundamental vocabulary of
"entitlement" and "accountability": double entry bookkeeping, the outlook,
really, of the bourgeois sytem. It seems to be false to what we know. In
a way it registers a bare legal minimum. If we were adversary lawyers
battling for opposite sides, I think these might be appropriate terms.
But surely our experience with our families, with our friends, with our
patients is--whether joy, whether love, whether growth and grace--is that
all these things accrue precisely when people realize that they are getting
more than their entitlement. The growth in the giver is when he is giving
more than he is strictly liable or accountable for. It is in that area
that the real growth occurs. When the child realizes that he is loved
beyond entitlement, beyond anything that you could put into a balanced
ledger of what you put in and take out, it is then that he feels called
upon also to give more than he is accountable for. Surely this vocabulary
is the vocabulary of a minimum--which is false to what we do at our best
and, normally, at our most intuitive.

Nagy: I think this is very much to the fundamental point, and I do agree that this is a base line. If this is violated, if you go on to say, "Let's have it this way forever, you give more and I receive more." At that point it becomes what I call ethical stagnation. At that point it has a fixed imbalance: now I exploit you; you always give me more than I am entitled to, and I always receive more.

This is a base line. I don't retreat from this basic ethical point; then I can add these other things to it.

But I wanted to make a point in relation to what Sam was saying, and it may bring us back to a practical illustration of what I am talking about: how to use this as a dynamic. A dying child comes to my mind. I have been in a number of situations in which the child has cancer--a girl of thirteen, let's say. I remember a very lovely girl already developing into young womanhood, and regretting that she will never become a mother because she knows she has to die in a few months of cancer. And her parents are (especially her mother is) completely broken by grief. The usual psychodynamic or psychological attitude would be that the child should receive from the parent, that the parent should be strengthened to give to the child, especially since the child is facing dying, and the parents should have resources to give more to the dying child.

I was thinking about this because I had to deal with this family in family therapy--it was some kind of family-based pediatric-based intervention with my help. What I came to, in my logic, was that the child now is more helped by my addressing myself to the child's accountability rather than her entitlement, even though the child is, in a way, entitled to more than anybody else. Here is a young life which will never grow to full maturity, which will have to stop in a miserable way in a few months. So the child is really the victim. But, I started to think, who is more deprived of resources--the child who is to die, or the parent whose young child is to die? And I started to think, "Maybe the parent is even more unable to give." So I started to work on this basis: Why not see what are the child's resources to help the grieving parents? And why not look on this as the main resource? And this worked! As I started to think whether this girl was sitting there in pain, I noticed that her mother was sitting there all morning, crying, and wouldn't be able to say anything. The nurses wanted to restrict visiting because the mother upset the child. I noticed that the child would say, "Mother, why don't you do some knitting or something?" So the child was already the one who was the resource, who wanted to direct the mother, to help the mother with her grief. So I started to capitalize on this aspect of the system: that its resources really lay in making use of the accountability of the dying child-- because if we had only looked at the entitlement there was nothing to do. "Alright, I sympathize with you; you have to die; that is horrible; how do you really feel about that?" "I also feel very bad about it." It is all passive. But if I say, instead, "But you will feel better if you can help your parents; in your dying days the knowledge will help that you can help your parents," it immediately makes sense to me. This provides for an active role. Here I can use something that can be done, even by the dying.

Then a nurse or social worker in the hospital said we should cut off the child completely from the parents, allow no visiting, and talk about

her school experience, and specifically made up dolls, and so on, to take
her mind off. . . . It wouldn't have made any sense. She would have been
just that much deeper into despair at not being able to do anything.
Whereas if she were made to help the visiting, grieving parents--at that
point she would be made to fight her predicament. She could do something.

So I come back to this because I think that the child is entitled,
the child is dependent and the parents should give. That's true. But I
think ordinary psychodynamic thinking underplays the other side--that the
child can also grow by accountability. The child would like to help the
parents--even a dying child would. I am just using this example as an
illustration of how accountability can be used as a resource.

Bloch: One of the things I would like to talk about, because I think it
gets to the issue of the relationship of larger and more powerful institutions to the kinds of things that we are talking about on the family level
is this.

I feel it is obligatory upon us to pay attention, for example, in
many of our teaching institutions, to how we treat each other. It is not
simply enough to treat our patients well and our students well. And,
in fact, we can't treat our patients and our students well, if we don't
treat each other well. And to be self-conscious about this--that is, to b
self-conscious about being fair and open, just in those general terms--is
important. The problem is, at least in my experience, that it is possible
to do this up to a certain size of an organization, and then the nature of
communication and the nature of the distribution of power and the economic

in the broadest and the most meticulous sense, begin to play out at that point. I feel this is the difficulty in translating into the next step up. I don't have any kind of an answer for that. I really feel dismayed by it, to be candid, but at least I would define the problem that way. There are human-sized institutions, and then there are inhuman-sized institutions. But I do think that at least we can maintain--it has to do with the face-to-face nature of the interaction. That is, as long as we interact face to face, we can be reasonably human with each other. You can know about forty or fifty people. It is not an abstract number. You can know about three layers in a hierarchy. That's it. A higher vertical thrust or a wider lateral size--that seems to require a whole different kind of ethical issue. That's the place where I feel baffled and, frankly, rather hopeless.

PART FOUR

Bloch: I really feel that I had no preconceptions at all for myself about what was going to happen here this week. And that was in keeping with the feeling that Henry had, that he wanted to bring together people whom he likes and who, he felt, shared some interests, in order to see what would happen if they addressed themselves to these enormously important and rather poorly articulated questions. And so we've done that. I've gotten a great deal out of this week in lots of ways, talking to people, listening to people, whom I would not otherwise have had a chance to. And I suspect that it may end up being rich and meaningful for me in ways that I can't yet calculate. It was also troublesome to me in that it was carried out on so many different levels of abstraction. . . . The task was so great that we had all the advantages of openness, but none of the closure, we might hope for. But that's perhaps a good thing. It gives us additional useful tension.

So I guess I'd like to suggest that one of the things we can do briefly is for those of us who are so inclined to say a little bit about what each was expecting when he came here and what he or she actually found. And, perhaps, also in a more formal way to answer: Is there some way in which this interest and attention to this problem--the nature of the relationship of ethics and something called "treatment," the "treatment enterprise," the "treatment apparatus,"--can improve for each person its ethical qualities?

Audience: I came here feeling totally depleted after working for one year on a treatment program for abused and neglected children and their families This last year I became very much aware of dilemmas in treatment. Whom do you treat when you have a parent, a middle-aged mother who has abused her children? The children come to you in treatment, and you have maybe eleven to thirteen-year-old girls who are about to give birth to another child. And the system does not lend itself to supporting the unborn child. To whom do you have the responsibility? How are you able to be sensitive, as Dr. Nagy was saying, to everybody concerned? And to the impacts that your treatment and your intervention have on all the family members? So I was really looking, in coming here, for an answer as to how to stay alive, as one of the members was saying. And I must say that there were some high-lights in the meeting. I was delighted to have a chance to hear more of Dr. Nagy's ethics of the dynamics of relationships. Even just raising the questions and realizing that everyone else experiences the dilemmas that I have experienced this last year is in a sense a help, because you feel that you are not alone.

I also felt that Dr. Seeley was sort of like John the Baptist, the voice crying in the wilderness, "Veni, veni." I felt I would like very much a copy of his paper. I think it would be challenging. I would like to show it to my students at the medical school. In that sense it was very helpful.

So I leave with as many questions as I had when I came. But I have a different feeling because I have been here.

Seeley: I feel tempted to respond. I deeply appreciated, in much the same way, some of the things that have happened: the obvious kindness and richness of the people, the setting in which this took place, the flexibility and openness of the program, the things we were forced to look at and might not otherwise have looked at. But I would have to add something that gives even greater force, and I do it reluctantly, to the "crying in the wilderness" effect. I would like to do this kind of thing again. I would like to do it many times. For either I am wrong on the leading contentions I made, or we are not serious.

If we are, as I suppose, at a moment, a very belated moment in the history of this civilization, well, either we can or cannot find a way to make the minor goods that we can each accomplish in our own lives accumulate into something that will make a better life (not leaving that to accident or to the hope that in some five thousand years a few people that we make better will somehow make something else better). Then, surely, the minimum response that we would make now, would be to find a way to so organize ourselves, so to remain in touch, so to differentiate ourselves from those who think otherwise and who are perfectly happy to use the same skills that we use to breathe life into people to strangle people. Surely we would now differentiate ourselves from these (and would find who are our allies, whatever profession, or whether they are professionals or not), who then, by necessity, at least pro tem, and in some formal sense, need to be seen as our opponents, if not our enemies. To do less than that is disgraceful; to do less than find a way (at whatever level we are working), as far as possible, to connect whatever good we do at that level with a good at the next most general level--so that when, for example, we strengthen someone psychologically at least we hope it does something to make a better family; and if we can make a better family, we take care to see that it doesn't stop there. We must take pains to see that it doesn't stop there, and that those families we deal with see that something about the way something else is organized is what makes it so hard to be a good family--so that there is always a link to a higher level, an ascending dialectic. That we take these problems seriously instead of leaving them to chance and to momentarily happy assemblages; that we take care of continuity. I am either wrong in my central contention, or, if we respond with less than that, then we are not serious.

Bloch: I remember many years ago when Crestwood Heights came out. I had the opportunity to review it for Scientific American. That led me to study the problem much more carefully than I would have. It seemed to me that you and your colleagues had a vision then, which is not, it seems to me, perfectly, seamlessly, continuous with the vision that you have expressed here. We were both a good deal younger then. But even then, it seemed to me that I was not sure how to proceed. That is, there are two kinds of problems associated with the view. One is that one of the least understood things, from my point of view, is the relationship between levels of system complexity. That is, that it is very, very hard, maybe intrinsically impossible, to know that, as a system of higher complexity is generated, how its characteristics will relate to the component systems that become its substructures. To put it in a very simple kind of way: it's impossible to know, from anything concerning the characteristics of sodium and chlorine, how salt will taste. There's no way to know that. I think it's

probably demonstrably unknowable. And I suspect that may be the problem
to which, in a considerably more complex way, you are addressing yourself.
Because I think that is at least one of the theoretic issues with which we
are dealing. And while I don't think a great deal is known about it, I
think there is something known about it. And it seems you can at best go
one level up. That is, we might be able to say, if we formed an organization here, something about the characteristics of how we would deal with
each other and whether we would have an ethically good organization.
How that would turn out if we became part of some other, more complex
organization (as inevitably occurs in society) is hard to say. At that
point it might be beyond us. In any case, I wanted to say that that issue,
which I think you are coming right at, is one which I'd like to put on the
agenda for the future. Can one, and how can one, do that? I don't mean in
any way to reduce the intensity of what you are saying, I think it moves
us all.

Coming back to Crestwood Heights--I think the good acts of the people
in that community and the good wishes and lofty motives were in part
related to producing the right managers for the enterprises of the commer-
cial and industrial world in which they live.

Why don't some other people talk in terms of things they may want to
put on the agenda for the future? How would one carry forward some of
these things that we're trying to understand or think about here? Or what
has this meant in a personal sense? I found what you had to say was very
moving.

Audience: I want to connect the two things if I can, because I've had difficulty assimilating some of the ideas [to Dr. Seeley]. I've been very charged by your ideas. But I don't move in the same ways you do. If I can cast you in the role of revolutionary, I'd like to do so. And I wonder if the role of revolutionary leaders is to start revolutions or to wake up the sleeping populace and to get things going in smaller places and in smaller ways. Because, if I read your fears correctly, it is too late. That was the title of your paper. I think the revolution won't take place in the way that you are asking for it to take place. I think the title accurately summarizes some of the things you're trying to encourage us to think about. Your last comment this morning was: "It can't happen in these small ways; there has to be some linkage of these forces of good." I'm an educator, primarily, and I believe in the force of education, and small ripples becoming wider, and small circles becoming interlinked with other circles and so on. I don't know the history of the world that well to know whether ideas can create movements in the way that you're asking for--these greater changes to take place in these major ways. I'm happy enough, maybe I'm complacent enough, to deal with my students, and to hope that when I raise these ethical issues with them that they'll then teach twenty-five hundred students some day who will raise the same issues in a more cogent and powerful way than I've raised them. So I'm much more able to wait and let it happen in small ways. And I'm wondering if that idea is compatible; if you find that to be totally at odds with your point of view.

Seeley: I find it seriously at odds with my point of view. Though, because of the ambiguities, I'd like to avoid revolutionary/counter-revolutionary dichotomies. Let me take a few things from your own field. (Let me also add that at or about the time of Crestwood Heights I indeed believed like you, though perhaps if I had been a bit more thoughtful, even then, I should have seen differently.)

Take something in your own field, intended as liberating in its intent, for example the development of the Binet tests of intelligence. One object was, not to lay upon children burdens which they couldn't bear. It was almost like trying to find a way to recognize the child's strength before you set him an athletic task or gave him a burden to carry, and not punishing him because he was small and couldn't carry the burden. So the test became a relative test of his capacity and that was the intended use of the intelligence test. What it turned out to be was something that, in general, permitted teachers to apply, with a better conscience, a more rigid screw upon the child, because now they "knew" what his capacity was, and they felt very righteous in making him live up to it and demanding this more rigidly. And then, in something that was not in their control because they were not united, they were not in command of either the resources of education, or the reproductive resources of education (by reproductive resources I mean teachers were not in control of the processes by which teachers were trained, by and large). The testing system became the parent of the "tracking" system.

Let me give you another illustration that might seem beautifully innocent. Not very long ago there was a serious attempt made, because

someone believed in it very deeply, to detect in advance "violence-prone
children." It's a rather dangerous idea in a way. But let's say "children
with a very low frustration threshold." And let's neglect for the moment
the oversight of context and whatever else is involved. But it was believed
you could detect the so-called "violence-proneness" early. Now, you can
take a very repressive view of that and say, "Well, of course they would
use that to suppress or repress such children or to change them by force,
by behavior modification." But let's not suppose that for the same reasons
as make me like to wipe out Henry's unfortunate side-effects of his drugs,
and say, "What would the situation be if the side effects were good?"--
because it would sharpen the problem. Let's assume that this successful
test was in the best of hands, and that we did detect which children would
have low frustration thresholds, and we were very kind towards them, and
put those with very low frustration thresholds in classes where they would
get special treatment, where the frustration level was very low. We would
again introduce a tracking system which we are now only throwing out of the
schools in the intelligence thing. And the whole process would turn out,
in effect, barring other safeguards, which are not intrinsic to nice
educators sitting down and hoping for ripple effects--it would again,
almost surely, result in a tracking system which would also turn out to be
a poverty and minority-separation system. I'm only describing. I'm not
asking the impossible--what you would designate as "the revolution,"
whether violence is involved or not, I do not want to predict and I do
not claim to know. And I do not ask the impossible. I ask only that
people see not merely the proximate effects of what they do, but the next
effects, and, if possible, the next effects. To see as far as the ultimate

effects--that's impossible; we would have to be gods. But I ask that at least people see, and take responsibility for acting as far as they can (and that does entail responsibility) to make sure that they have that much control, that they are not really powerless, and cannot be simply used as tools, so that one problem becomes fashionable and then another, in what is, I believe, in effect, nothing much more then, than a diversionary spectacle. But, I ask that at every point, whenever one is working, we become connected (like a bucket brigade) so that those of us who are working doing therapy with individuals are at least concerned with families; and those working with families are at least concerned with what puts certain classes of families in a position where it is sure that eighty percent of them must undergo unbearable strains, not because they don't know how to run a family, but because circumstances are such that other pressures make it almost impossible for them to operate.

And I ask that those who see one piece would connect with those who can see the next piece, and at least that we stay together and recognize who of us are in that operation, even given the division of labor. None of us can understand everything. But if we knew who we were, and if we were together, and if we made sure that someone was attending to every part of the task by these linkages, and when all knew who was doing or undoing what, and doing otherwise--then I would have a feeling that we were beginning to be serious.

Bloch: I have two phrases which keep recurring in my mind. One of them is the old one: "The road to hell is paved with good intentions"--long known, not a discovery at all. But the other one is, I think, Schrödinger:

"Life feeds on negative entropy." In effect, at any level, what differen-
tiates the animate from the inanimate is the fact that the movement towards
entropy, towards increasing randomness, is defeated by organization and by
creating structure. Clearly, if there is a dividing point between the
animate and the inanimate, it is on the line where the thrust towards
entropy is defeated. Now it seems to me that that is what we are talking
about. And we are talking always, at any level, about the fact that there
is a price for this. We, as humans, steal negative entropy from plants
(that's a decent way to steal it). But, to use Erikson's phrase, we
"pseudo-speciate" our colleagues--which means that we make them edible,
we can eat our colleagues, because they now become another species.

I think that what you are describing is a recurrent and inevitable
and unavoidable fact: that with consciousness comes the awareness of this
aspect of the psychobiological world. That's like railing at gravitation.
All I'm saying--I'm trying to give a very quick shorthand summary of why
this happens--but I think you are always going to find yourself in this
situation, which may be a good place to be.

Nagy: I would like to get into something that Don is saying, because something comes into my mind about this conference and about some of the
directions.

Schrödinger's negative entropy, and life and structure building--that
may be the kind of structure that we are perhaps examining here. In my
terms again, what we are asking about is the trustworthiness of the whole
helping industry--from both sides. Now we can take one side only, and
say, "Let's be consumer advocates unilaterally, and let's find the rotten

doctors. . .you know, let's do our own thing. And yet they are being
trusted, and they are not really being trusted, because they are not trustworthy. So if we just make the health care industry more accountable,
answerable, unilaterally, so that they deserve more trust because they are
more concerned and fair and so on, then really we do our job."

On the other side, we might say (and I was really trying to put in
this other notion) that, maybe real trustworthiness is a dialogue of
answerability: that somehow the underdog is being helped not just by
condescendingly being protected--"You don't know enough; those who are in
power should be more concerned." But that, also linked with that, there
should be some answerability placed on the consumers too. For instance,
I was thinking of producing children in a more responsible way, or whatever--
which is another side. That we could help, maybe, trustworthiness, by
finding how everybody could be answerable in a better way.

So there would be two ways of looking at the problem--the traditional,
liberal-progressive way would be simply taking the unilateral consumer-
advocacy position. But I wonder if that is short-changing the consumers.

Lennard: I don't think that this is our position. We are most concerned
that physicians aren't encouraging people to be responsible for their wellbeing and health, and are not encouraging all efforts where persons take
an active role in being responsible, informing themselves, and knowing as
much as possible about their health. I don't think anyone here is really
making unilateral accusations, that we are only holding the doctors or the
family therapists accountable. Everyone is responsible!

Nagy: But that is different from really defining those areas where, as consumers, we can be more accountable. It is different from saying, "Take a more active part in that which the experts are doing so that you cannot be fooled." That is very different from a broad exploration of all your contribution to what eventually becomes an ecological mess. That is a broader scope.

Seeley: When I said that you would have to find other allies and a different material base, that's what I meant. There is no answer unless you find a mass alliance and regard yourself as a part of that alliance, and unless you find a base that is not mediated and controlled by the State, which has a different set of interests. That's what I mean about being serious. The problems are so connected that, ripple effects or no ripple effects, at the best and the happiest, the ripple effects are allowed to play themselves out in some corners of an exemplary school here or an exemplary school there, which, on the whole, permits an educational system to continue that really truncates children and teaches them to separate thought from feeling and action and commitment.

Until we are theoretically clear on this as organizational fact and committed to stay with each other and with the vast alliance that we can win to our side--not talking to them from some vast distance up here, but recognizing that they are more like us than not--until something like that happens, I think we really are doing nothing but cosmetic work.

Bloch: We have to find a way to do that, that will not, in a few more moments of history, produce exactly the thing that we are against.

I think one of the things that crossed my desk recently that appalled me. . .I got a communication from a major American School of Medicine in which continuing medical education is now offering a course on Depression, and the course is supported by one of the major drug companies. A beautifully packaged, highly glossy collection, in which big television programs are being produced, a collection of documents, teaching materials; and the course is given for credit under the continuing medical education program.

What's the particular horror? The idea of continuing medical education is, on the whole a good idea. The doctors should not, when they get out of medical school--because we know that they stop learning, most of them--limit what they know to a few things. And it's a good idea to do this. But if you do this you have to police it. Because you have both to reward them--give them credits, physician-recognition awards, there's a whole apparatus for doing that--and also you have to prod them from behind, in addition to putting the carrot out front. You have the stick in back, which is that they aren't going to get re-licensed if they don't do that. So this is going to get doctors re-educated.

So who jumps in on this? Two big power groups--the drug companies on the one hand, and a big medical school on the other hand. And what are they doing? They pick something which, maybe, is part of the human condition, or occasionally is a disease, called "despression"; and now they are pushing a course. And you can be damned sure of what that course is selling--it's selling drugs. Bing, bing, bing; one, two, three; good idea, good idea, good idea. And then!

It seems possible that the ethical issues and the structural issues maybe cannot be approached. I don't know if they can be. But to follow it up by the usual approach which is to build a new mass organization-- I don't know.

The way I would generalize is to talk about what I do try to talk about; which is built-in disequilibrators. That is, that somehow anti-stability, anti-system, anti-negative entropy subsystems are built into every system that we are a part of. That is, for me, a little glimmer of a way to think about this. I think those allies are those people that will unsettle us, will keep us alive (to use the other way of describing it) to those experiences.

Springer: Both of us [the Springers] enjoyed the sessions, because we hav been confronted with openness and the possibility to discuss from points of view different from those we are used to in Vienna. Also we have been confronted with teachers with a critical mind. So I could say the future has already begun here because we see teachers who are that critical. I have been influenced by Lennard's work, without knowing him before, by reading books by him in Vienna.

In Vienna, and I think in Germany too, the situation is much more closed. The discussion about ethical questions goes on, but among the younger people. And we don't know if they will ever be powerful enough to be teachers. Because to be a teacher in medicine or philosophy in Vienna is a very powerful position since there are very few Chairs. There have been times when you couldn't speak about "dialectics" in philosophy because "dialectics" was thought to be synonymous with "dialectic material-ism," and, therefore, you would be thought to be a Communist, and then you would not be able to get a Chair. That is the situation with us.

That is the most impressive thing that we learnt here: that you can criticize each other and still have a positive relationship; that you can fight at a round-table and then speak again together at the dinner table.

Also we have seen that one matter could change to another matter, and there always was some relationship between the issues and between the people who spoke about them. It was a group, and a beautiful group in a way that not every person had to share the opinions of all the others.

A NOTE ON LOCATION AND

FORMAT

The Conference on ETHICS OF HEALTH CARE was held
in the Ateneo Veneto in Venice, Italy in July 1977. Venice
is a fitting site for a conference examining the problems
associated with a proliferation of health care technologies and therapeutic techniques. Venice more than any
other city has resisted, though not wholly escaped the most
severe effects of modern technology. Its citizens still
relish the joy and drama of everyday life and human related-
ness.

The format of the Conference is closely patterned
after those organized for the Josiah Macy Jr. Foundation
by Frank Freemont Smith -- which allowed for a great deal
of discussion, even if not always relevant -- and retained
the flavor of the spontaneous interchange in its conference
publications. In editing the Conference proceedings, we
have omitted and revised as little as feasible, though more
than we had hoped initially. Publication costs forced us
to omit a lengthy paper by John Seeley prepared for a
special evening session. Copies of the paper are available
by writing to the publisher.

ABOUT THE PARTICIPANTS

Samuel T. Anderson, M.D. is a Psychiatrist in Greenbrae,
California and has been affiliated with
the Marin Psychiatric Foundation.

Donald A. Bloch, M.D. directs the Ackerman Institute for
Family Therapy, serves as the editor of
Family Process and is author of Techni-
ques of Family Psychotherapy.

Ivan Boszormenyi-Nagi, M.D. has been affiliated with the
Eastern Pennsylvania Psychiatric Insti-
tute, Jefferson and Hahnemann Medical
Colleges and is the author of Intensive
Family Therapy and Invisible Loyalties.

Ruth Cooperstock   is with the Addiction Research Foundation of Ontario and has been a consult-
ant to the Non-Medical Use of Drugs
Directorate. She edited Social Aspects
of Psychotropic Drugs.

Suzanne Crowhurst-Lennard, Ph.D. has been affiliated with
the University of California at Berkeley,
SUNY at New Paltz and SUNY at Purchase.
She is the author of Explorations in the
Meaning of Architecture.

Henry L. Lennard, Ph.D. has been affiliated with the University of California at San Francisco,
School of Medicine and with Columbia
University, Center for Policy Research
and Yeshiva University. He is the author of Patterns in Human Interaction
and Mystification and Drug Misuse.

Philip Sapir   past President of the William T. Grant
Foundation, has been affiliated with the
National Institute of Mental Health, the
Albert Einstein College of Medicine and
the National Institute of Child Health
and Human Development.

John R. Seeley, Ph.D. has been affiliated with the Center
for Democratic Institutions, Santa
Barbara, the University of Toronto, the

University of California at Los Angeles and the Charles R. Drew Postgraduate Medical School. He is the author of Crestwood Heights and the Americanization of the Unconscious.

Harley C. Shands, M.D. is chairman of the Department of Psychiatry at Roosevelt Hospital, and has been affiliated with the University of North Carolina, Downstate Medical Center and Columbia University. He is the author of The War with Words and Speech as Instruction.

Alfred Springer, M.D. directs the Ludwig Boltzman Institut for Addiction Research in Vienna and is the publisher and editor of the Wiener Zeitschrift fuer Suchtforschung.

Marianne Springer-Kremser, M.D. has been affiliated with the Department of Psychosomatic Medicine, Gynecological Clinic, and Institut fuer Tiefenpsychologie and Psychotherapie, both at the University of Vienna.